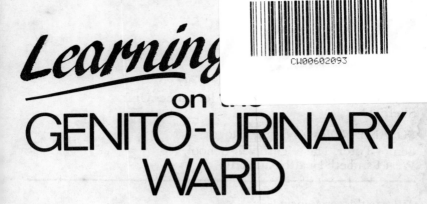

Learning
on the
GENITO-URINARY WARD

Rosalind Boddington
SRN, DN(London), RCNT, PGCEA

Tutor in Genito-urinary Surgery,
The Nightingale School,
St Thomas's Hospital,
London

HODDER AND STOUGHTON
LONDON SYDNEY AUCKLAND TORONTO

LEARNING TO CARE SERIES

General Editors

JEAN HEATH, MED, BA, SRN, SCM, CERT ED
English National Board Learning Resources Unit,
Sheffield

SUSAN E NORMAN, SRN, DNCERT, RNT
Senior Tutor, The Nightingale School,
West Lambeth Health Authority

Titles in this series include:
Learning to Care in the A&E Department
G JONES
Learning to Care in the Theatre
K NIGHTINGALE
Learning to Care in Midwifery
J ALEXANDER

ISBN 0 340 41308 5

First published 1987
Copyright © 1987 R Boddington

Typeset in 10/11pt Trump Mediaeval by
Rowland Phototypesetting Ltd, Bury St Edmunds, Suffolk

Printed in Great Britain for Hodder and Stoughton Educational,
a division of Hodder and Stoughton Ltd, Mill Road, Dunton Green,
Sevenoaks, Kent, TN13 2YD, by Richard Clay Ltd, Bungay, Suffolk

EDITORS' FOREWORD

In most professions there is a traditional gulf between theory and its practice, and nursing is no exception. The gulf is perpetuated when theory is taught in a theoretical setting and practice is taught by the practitioner.

This inherent gulf has to be bridged by students of nursing, and publication of this series is an attempt to aid such bridge building.

It aims to help relate theory and practice in a meaningful way whilst underlining the importance of the person being cared for.

It aims to introduce students of nursing to some of the more common problems found in each new area of experience in which they will be asked to work.

It aims to de-mystify some of the technical language they will hear, putting it in context, giving it meaning and enabling understanding.

PREFACE

The aim of this nursing text is to introduce you to aspects of genito-urinary nursing, using a care-study approach. The emphasis is on practical aspects of care in order that it can be useful to you on the ward, helping you to link theory with practice.

It is important for you to develop the skills of problem-solving, to understand the rationale behind the care that you give and to be aware of current research and development, in order that you can use it to the benefit of your patients.

The names used are fictitious and do not refer to actual people. The feminine gender is used throughout when referring to nurses, without prejudice to male nurses and purely for convenience.

Acknowledgements. I am grateful to all my friends and colleagues for their support and advice and to my parents, especially my father for typing the manuscript. Most particularly, this book would not have been possible without the patience and encouragement of Michael, to whom I owe so much.

CONTENTS

Introduction

On arriving on the genito-urinary ward you will find that many aspects of the nursing care will be familiar to you – for example, you will probably have cared for patients with urinary catheters or incontinence during previous ward experiences.

Patients of all ages who have dysfunction of their urinary system find their problem very embarrassing. Such symptoms as incontinence or frequency of micturition have serious implications for many patients attempting to carry on normal everyday life. As a member of the nursing team here, you will require particular skill and ability to demonstrate empathy and understanding, as well as sound communication skills. An awareness of the ways in which people of different cultures respond to such problems is also important.

The age group of your patients may vary, and while many may be young or middle-aged, the majority will probably be elderly. Many skills you have already mastered in caring for these age groups will be valuable to you here.

Perhaps one of the main points to consider when caring for older patients in the genito-urinary ward is that they may suffer from a number of other disorders or illnesses which might affect their hospital stay, treatment and subsequent recovery. Some of your patients, for example, may have cardiac failure, chronic airways disease, or arthritis. They may also have difficulties with hearing or vision which may affect their progress while in your care.

There may be a preponderance of male patients in the ward, as one of the most common genito-urinary problems is that of enlargement of the prostate gland – a problem for many older gentlemen.

The average length of stay of the patients you will meet will vary considerably – from an overnight stay for a patient undergoing an investigative procedure, to several weeks for those having major surgery. You should always remember that whatever problems your patients have, most will be anxious about coming into hospital, and your approach to them can do a great deal to allay their anxiety (Franklin 1974).

Some of the patients you meet here will have malignant disease of the genito-urinary tract, for example, carcinoma of the kidney, bladder or testis. You may have cared for other patients with malignancies, and while all these disorders vary in their progress and outcome, many of the skills and principles of care that you have learned will assist you. You will probably have learned the important points about general pre- and post-operative care, and so this book will deal with aspects of care which are more specific to the particular specialty.

In this ward you will have a particular opportunity to develop your knowledge and understanding of catheters, as many of your patients will require them. There are many reasons why your patients may be catheterised, for instance:

1 To relieve obstruction or blockage of the urinary system.
2 Incontinence of urine.
3 To obtain accurate measurement of urine output.
4 Following trauma or injury to the urinary system.

A Foley catheter

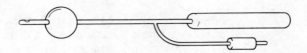

5 To promote healing following urinary surgery.
6 To enable investigation of the urinary tract to be performed.
7 Following lower abdominal surgery when micturition may be difficult.

Perhaps, in your previous experience, you have encountered one type of catheter used for basic urinary drainage (e.g. a Foley catheter). You will learn here about different types of catheters and the rationale behind their selection. Many of your patients will have undergone surgery to the urinary tract, and the choice of catheter will be relevant to that.

Each of the chapters in this book will highlight patients' problems that you may encounter on this ward. *It is important, however, that you see all patients as individual people, and not merely as one of a number with similar problems.*

Following general information and a nursing history of the patient, the chapters will present aspects of nursing care based upon a problem-solving approach. Therefore, particular problems (both actual and potential) will be identified, as they would be on the ward, by the nurse and the patient together. The nursing care will then be described with the rationale, as it is important for you to understand why you give the care that you do.

As the book is designed to help you primarily with the delivery of care, you will need a sound knowledge of the basic structure and function of the genito-urinary tract. You may already have studied this, but revision will be helpful as it will enable you to understand much more easily the problems of your patients.

Before moving on to the next chapter, ensure that you can draw a basic diagram of the urinary tract, to include kidneys, ureters, bladder and urethra. You should understand the male reproductive system and its relationship to the urinary system, and be able to explain briefly the physiology of micturition.

To assist you with this, and throughout the book, there will be a list of references and further reading at the ends of the chapters. In case of difficulty in finding these particular references, talk to the staff in the nurse education centre. You should find similar relevant reading in your nursing library. In addition, there will also be questions through which you can consolidate your knowledge, and, where appropriate, additional points for you to consider.

FURTHER READING

Ross, J. S. & Wilson, K. J. W. 1981. *Foundations of Anatomy and Physiology*. 5th Ed. Edinburgh & London: Churchill Livingstone.

Gibson, J. 1981. *Modern Physiology and Anatomy for Nurses*. 2nd Ed. Oxford: Blackwell Scientific Publications.

Jacob, S. W., Francone, C. A. & Lossow, W. J. 1978. *Structure and Function in Man*. 4th Ed. London: W. B. Saunders Company.

Hewitt, F. S. 1981. Communication skills – The nurse & the patient. *Nursing Times* (series from January to October 28th 1981).

Franklin, B. L. 1974. *Patient Anxiety on Admission to Hospital*. London: RCN.

2 Caring for patients with urinary incontinence

HISTORY

Nursing Mrs Peters who has stress incontinence

Mrs Gladys Peters is a 64-year-old lady who lives with her husband in a first-floor flat. She has seven children who are all married and living locally. She is an active member of her local over-60's club, and she and her husband organise many trips and outings for the members. She also works three mornings per week in a local launderette.

For approximately two years she has been troubled by stress incontinence. She finds this both uncomfortable and embarrassing, not only when going out socially, but also at home. Although her husband is very understanding about the problem, she feels it is beginning to cause a rift between them as she becomes more reluctant to go out for long periods of time. She therefore visits her GP, and following an Outpatient referral, her admission for investigation is arranged.

Stress incontinence is loss of urine which occurs with sudden increases in intra-abdominal pressure, i.e. laughing, coughing and physical exertion, e.g. lifting. Most commonly affects women who have had multiple pregnancies and may be overweight.

Incontinence occurs under stress due to relaxation or weakness of the pelvic floor musculature, which results in the urethra becoming shortened and the posterior angle of the bladder neck reduced.

INITIAL NURSING CARE

Mrs Peters is welcomed to the ward and shown to her bed by Margaret Jones, the ward nurse. After showing her the facilities and introducing her to patients in the adjacent beds,

The muscles of the pelvic floor. (a) Normal pelvic floor musculature (b) The pelvic floor musculature in stress incontinence

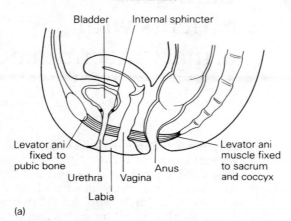

(a)

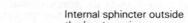

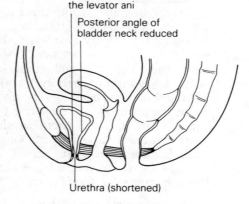

(b)

Margaret leaves Mrs Peters to unpack, before returning to obtain a full nursing history.

As Mrs Peters finds it difficult and embarrassing to discuss her problem, Margaret makes every attempt to show concern and understanding. She takes Mrs Peters to a private place within the ward so that she may feel more at ease when giving details of the extent of her problem.

Mrs Peters tells Margaret that she finds it embarrassing to explain things to someone of similar age to her own grand-daughter. Margaret reassures her that she has cared for other patients with similar problems and does appreciate her apprehension.

Mrs Peters also expresses concern about the investigations which the doctor has planned for her, as she did not feel able to ask many questions in the clinic because of her embarrassment. Margaret explains that the doctor

An example of an incontinence chart

Name _____

Chart the *volume passed* at the appropriate time. Tick if wet

Date	6/10		7/10		8/10		9/10		10/10		11/10		12/10	
	Volume passed	wet	Volume passed	wet	Volume passed	wet	Volume passed	wet	Volume passed	wet	Volume passed	wet	Volume passed	wet
Time														
12 MN														
01^{00}														
02^{00}														
03^{00}														
04^{00}														
05^{00}														
06^{00}														
07^{00}														
08^{00}														
09^{00}														
10^{00}														
11^{00}														
12^{00}														
13^{00}														
14^{00}														
15^{00}														
16^{00}														
17^{00}														
18^{00}														
19^{00}														
20^{00}														
21^{00}														
22^{00}														
23^{00}														
Total														

will need to know the degree and frequency of the incontinence, and that he will explain any tests in detail. She reassures her that she and the other nurses will ensure that she is fully prepared for all investigations. (Refer now to the Nursing Care Plans for Mrs Peters.)

RETURNING HOME

Mrs Peters returns home having established a routine for her exercises. They are written down for her should she wish to refer to the instructions, although she assures Margaret that they are imprinted on her memory.

As it is important to monitor progress and to give her encouragement and support, she is given an appointment to return every two weeks initially, then extending to every four weeks. In the clinic she will have a vaginal examination as this will indicate the degree of pelvic floor control, and hence improvement. She is advised that some positive results should be seen in 8–12 weeks, and that maximum benefit may take 6–9 months to achieve. It is important that Mrs Peters is prepared for this, as undue disappointment may affect her motivation to continue.

Having included her husband in discussions, he takes an interest in the programme and his encouragement will be a great support to her. All the indications are that she will be very successful in dealing with her incontinence in this way.

Nursing Care Plan for Mrs Peters

ACTUAL PROBLEM	NURSING CARE AND RATIONALE	EVALUATION
She is embarrassed about her incontinence, and particularly about any offensive odour which may be associated with it.	Margaret advises Mrs Peters to continue wearing a pad as she is used to it, and as this gives her a feeling of security. She explains that pads can be changed frequently, (and gives her adequate supplies and disposal bags). This, together with attention to personal hygiene, will minimise the risk of offensive odours, as Margaret points out to Mrs Peters, urine which is freshly passed carries very little odour.	Frequent changing of wet pads and good personal hygiene ensure minimal embarrassment for Mrs Peters and she is less concerned about odour.
Mrs Peters is concerned that she will be rejected by her husband and family.	Margaret encourages Mrs Peters to include her husband in discussions about her care. In this way they will both come to understand how this type of incontinence has occurred and how it can be treated.	Although concerned at first, Mrs Peters is pleased that her husband is included, and he is very interested and willing to co-operate in any way that will help her. As a result she is much less anxious.
Mrs Peters is worried about the extent of her incontinence and what treatment will be offered to her.	Margaret explains that in order to offer the correct treatment, an accurate record of the incontinence needs to be made on a special chart (an incontinence chart) to assess its severity.	Although, initially, Mrs Peters feels this is rather humiliating, with support and encouragement and good explanation she is able to appreciate its importance, and is pleased to participate in her care in some way.

9

Nursing Care Plan for Mrs Peters

ACTUAL PROBLEM	NURSING CARE AND RATIONALE	EVALUATION
Mrs Peters is worried about the investigation known as a *micturating cystometrogram* which she is to undergo to assess further her bladder function. Although the doctor has explained, she is apprehensive.	Margaret reassures her that this investigation will be carried out with concern for her dignity. She is able to arrange for the nurse who will be in the department at the time to visit her and discuss the test so as to reduce her anxiety.	Although it can be an embarrassing investigation, Mrs Peters is able to have this performed with the minimum of problems, helped by the fact that she knew the staff in the department. The results of this and other tests are encouraging, and Mrs Peters is advised that her incontinence will not require surgery, but can be relieved by pelvic floor exercises.

A micturating cystometrogram (MCM) is the main investigation in urodynamic studies (i.e. the study of pressure and flow in the lower urinary tract). Two catheters are passed into the bladder after the patient has voided. One catheter fills the bladder, the other measures bladder pressure. A third catheter is passed into the rectum, and measures general abdominal pressure. The bladder is filled rapidly with saline (0.9%), and the patient states (a) when the first desire to pass urine is felt, and (b) when the maximum volume for comfort has been reached. The filling catheter is then removed, and the patient is asked to stand and to increase abdominal pressure (e.g. by coughing). The patient then empties the bladder via a flow meter which measures the rate of urinary flow. Throughout the procedure, any incontinence is noted. This investigation requires the staff involved to explain everything fully both before and during the procedure to minimise the patient's embarrassment. Anxious and distressed patients may also produce inaccurate results.

Mrs Peters Learns to Perform Pelvic Floor Exercises

ACTUAL PROBLEM	NURSING CARE AND RATIONALE	WHAT DO PELVIC FLOOR EXERCISES INVOLVE?	EVALUATION
Mrs Peters has to learn how to perform pelvic floor exercises.	An exercise programme is drawn up with the help of the physiotherapist. Margaret explains to Mrs Peters that the muscles of the pelvic floor are like a hammock suspended between the front and back of the body. In her case these muscles have lost tone after the birth of seven children, and no longer exert tight control over the opening of the bladder. It is important for Mrs Peters to understand this as, being well-informed, she will feel more involved in her care and may be encouraged to work at her exercises.	1. Interruption of the urinary flow in midstream each time the patient passes urine. 2. Contraction of the pelvic floor muscles for a period of several seconds, 4–6 times every waking hour of every day. (This can be linked to daily activities.)	Mrs Peters is pleased not to be having an operation, and is very committed to improving her incontinence by her exercises.

(Now turn back to p. 8).

Nursing Mr Gibson with incontinence secondary to Parkinson's Disease

Mr George Gibson is a 76-year-old gentleman who is married, and lives with his wife in a cottage with a large garden, situated in a small village. Mr Gibson has had Parkinson's Disease for 10 years. He has become gradually more incapacitated by his illness, although he is still able to help his wife with some household chores and a little gardening. His main difficulty at present is a three-month history of incontinence which has been a particular problem at night or when going out.

Mr and Mrs Gibson have no family, and Mrs Gibson, at 70 years of age, finds it difficult at times to manage to run the home and to give her husband increasing help. The recent months have been a distressing and difficult time for both of them.

Mrs Gibson has encouraged her husband to use the downstairs toilet frequently during the day, which has helped to prevent incontinence although he still experiences some dribbling of urine. Due to the problem at night, however, they have had to sleep in separate beds and she has found the extra washing difficult to cope with.

The GP knows Mr Gibson well and arranges for admission to hospital for investigation and advice in the hope of improving the couple's quality of life.

Parkinson's Disease A degenerative disorder of the basal ganglia and nuclei in the upper brain stem (important for the complex reflexes enabling voluntary micturition). There is an imbalance of cerebral neurotransmitters with a relative deficiency of dopamine. Symptoms are poor movement, tremor and rigidity. The bladder's ability to empty effectively is often impaired.

INITIAL NURSING CARE

Mr and Mrs Gibson arrive on the ward after a long journey. They are welcomed by Margaret, the ward nurse, who makes them some tea and shows them to Mr Gibson's bed. He has been allocated a bed near the toilet so that he is able to reach it easily when required.

A nursing history is obtained by talking with Mr and Mrs Gibson. He has difficulties with speech because of his Parkinson's Disease, but is also embarrassed to talk about his problem.

Margaret observes that they are both very tired, not only as a result of their journey, but also because of Mr Gibson's problem. They are aware that his general condition will not improve, and are worried about how they will cope in the future. Margaret reassures them that there are a number of ways in which some of their difficulties can be alleviated, and that every effort will be made to improve their quality of life.

She is careful to obtain full details of Mr Gibson's daily routine in order to make his stay as comfortable as possible. (Now refer to the Nursing Care Plan for Mr Gibson.)

Application of a penile sheath

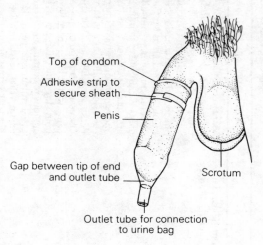

Top of condom

Adhesive strip to secure sheath

Penis

Gap between tip of end and outlet tube

Scrotum

Outlet tube for connection to urine bag

Nursing Care Plan for Mr Gibson

PROBLEM	NATURE	NURSING CARE AND RATIONALE	EVALUATION
Actual	Incontinence of urine, particularly at night.	Margaret explains to Mr Gibson that to assess his problem accurately a record must be made of the frequency with which he urinates or is incontinent. She records each occasion on the incontinence chart as Mr Gibson finds difficulty in doing so himself because of his Parkinsonian tremor. She provides Mr Gibson with a urinal, as one reason for his incontinence has been slow toileting due to his Parkinson's Disease. Margaret discusses with him the use of pads and pants which he has been wearing at home for protection, and as he is anxious to continue with these to avoid embarrassing episodes, she ensures that he has an adequate supply. She checks that he has the nurse-call button within easy reach so that he can summon assistance at any time.	A pattern of incontinence is seen from the chart which Margaret keeps. Use of the urinal is successful in reducing Mr Gibson's problem in the daytime. At night time, however, it is not helpful as he is unable to use it in bed, and this is, therefore, still of concern to him.

Actual	Mr Gibson has excoriated skin around the scrotum, penis and perineum due to incontinence.	Margaret ensures that Mr Gibson is able to change pads whenever necessary to minimise skin damage by pads saturated with urine. He is assisted with personal hygiene to keep his skin clean and dry, and offered hoist baths. As wet pads are now mainly a problem at night, Margaret suggests to Mr Gibson that he uses a *penile sheath*, attached to a drainage bag at night, thus avoiding the need for pads at all. She spends considerable time explaining its use to him and to his wife, and applies one for him to try.	Mr Gibson's skin improves and is no longer excoriated. The use of the sheath ensures that no wet pads damage his skin at night, and his sleep is not disturbed.
Actual	Embarrassment at the amount of assistance Mr Gibson requires with his problem.	Margaret encourages Mr Gibson to be as independent as possible in order to maintain his dignity. She ensures that he has privacy when using the urinal.	Mr Gibson's embarrassment is diminished by the consideration for his dignity, and as he gains confidence in the nursing staff.
Potential	Dehydration, as Mr Gibson has become reluctant to drink because of his incontinence.	Margaret explains to him that he should drink between one and two litres of fluid per 24 hours. This will prevent electrolyte imbalance caused by dehydration (which might make him confused). It will also ensure that he does not have to endure an unpleasant feeling of thirst. If his fluids are restricted resulting in the urinary tract being infrequently flushed through, he may also be susceptible to urinary tract infection.	Mr Gibson maintains the required fluid intake, thus avoiding any complications. He also feels more confident about this because of the improvement in his continence.

The penile sheath for incontinence is a soft latex sleeve which fits over the penis and allows urine to drain into a collection bag. It may be used by men with moderate or severe incontinence, and also where frequency or urgency make toiletting a problem. It is manufactured in a number of sizes. A sheath is usually applied to clean, dry skin using a fixation strip halfway along the penis. This should not be wrapped around too tightly in order to avoid constriction. Long pubic hair should be trimmed. Ensuring that the foreskin is not retracted, the sheath is unrolled for approximately 2 cm (which is the required gap between the end of the penis and the beginning of the outlet tube to provide a small reservoir), and then unrolled over the penis. The sheath should be checked to ensure that it is not causing constriction. Initially, it should be changed daily and the skin inspected. Once found to be suitable, it may remain *in situ* for up to three days. If the patient is not dextrous, he may require assistance to apply the sheath.

RETURNING HOME

Mr and Mrs Gibson are very pleased with the improvement in Mr Gibson's continence. They will continue with the use of the urinal in the daytime and the sheath at night and when going out (as it can then be connected to a leg drainage bag under the trousers).

Mrs Gibson has participated in her husband's care throughout, and has been shown how to help fit the sheath, as Mr Gibson is unable to manage this alone because of his Parkinson's Disease.

Margaret ensures that Mrs Gibson feels confident about this by discussing all the procedures once more before they leave. She explains that the District Nurse will call twice weekly, and that the GP will arrange prescriptions for supplies of sheaths.

As Mr Gibson relies on his wife to a greater extent now than ever, the Medical Social Worker is able to arrange for a home help to come three mornings per week to relieve Mrs Gibson's workload of shopping and housework.

Mr and Mrs Gibson feel that the problem is now under control, and are relieved to be resuming their lives together at home with what they consider to be an improvement in their quality of life.

TEST YOURSELF

1 What were the possible causes of Mrs Peters' stress incontinence?
2 How would you explain a micturating cystometrogram?
3 How could Mrs Peters be encouraged to carry out pelvic floor exercises?
4 What are the important aspects of skin care for incontinent patients?
5 How was the application of a penile sheath explained to Mr and Mrs Gibson?
6 What did both patients feel about their dependence upon nurses and others in coping with incontinence?

FURTHER READING

Blannin, J. 1984. Assessment of the incontinent patient. *Nursing* (2nd series), No. 29, September 1984. London: Medical Education.
Blannin, J. *et al.* 1986. Continence promotion. *Nursing* (3rd series), supplement to Issue 10, October 1986. London: Baillière Tindall.
Harrison, S. 1975. Physiotherapy in the treatment of stress incontinence. *Nursing Mirror*, **141**(2), 52–53.
Mandelstam, D. 1980. *Incontinence and Its Management*. Beckenham: Croom Helm.
Norton, C. 1986. *Nursing for Continence*. Bucks: Beaconsfield Publishers Ltd.

3 Caring for patients with indwelling catheters

Multiple sclerosis is a degenerative neuromuscular disease resulting from demyelination of the nerve fibres. It is progressive, with periods of exacerbation and remission. Nerve pathway damage can affect the cortical centre controlling micturition and the reflexes in the spinal cord and thus disrupt bladder function.

Nursing Mrs Green who requires a permanent indwelling catheter

Mrs Green is a 37-year-old mother of two children aged 10 years and 12 years. Her husband is a postman. Seven years ago she was diagnosed as having multiple sclerosis. Mrs Green is able to walk very little now, spending most of her time in a wheelchair.

The family have moved to a bungalow which has been specially adapted in order that Mrs Green can be as independent as possible, and care for her family in the same way as if she were completely fit. Unfortunately, she has now developed unpleasant urinary symptoms with which she can no longer cope. She has frequency and urgency of micturition, and – most embarrassing and distressing – occasional incontinence.

Micturition

Frequency of micturition
This is a disturbing symptom for patients. It results in a frequent desire to micturate – often for small amounts of urine. It may be caused by: inflammation of bladder (e.g. cystitis); increased urine volume due to increased fluid intake; inability of the bladder to empty properly; the effects of some drugs.

Urgency of micturition
This is a feeling of an immediate need to micturate if incontinence is to be avoided. It may be a symptom of inflammation of the bladder, or a neurological disorder.

Mrs Green is admitted for assessment, although the doctor has discussed with her in detail, in the clinic, that she may require a permanent catheter.

INITIAL NURSING CARE

Mrs Green arrives in the ward having travelled by ambulance. Her husband has remained at home to look after the children. The ward nurse, Margaret, welcomes her and shows her around the ward, pointing out the toilets which accommodate patients who are confined to wheelchairs. She helps her to unpack her belongings and get undressed. Whilst doing this, Mrs Green expresses concern to Margaret about her family, and how they will manage while she is in hospital. Margaret arranges with the ward sister for the Medical Social Worker to visit and discuss some possible arrangements with her.

Mrs Green's main anxiety, however, is her urinary problem, which, as she is confined to a wheelchair, she finds both socially and psychologically distressing – socially, because she is reluctant to go out, being unable to reach the toilet quickly and easily; and psychologically, because she feels embarrassed and humiliated, and is concerned that it is destroying her family life.

Margaret explains that Mrs Green will undergo investigations before final decisions are made, and explains the importance of recording the exact times at which she passes urine, and the volume passed.

Mrs Green is able to participate by recording this information herself, and this may help her to feel that she is contributing to her care. This chart will help to assess the extent of the problem.

Mrs Green has been told that she will have a micturating cystometrogram (see p. 10) to assess further her bladder function. Although the doctor has outlined the procedure, Margaret explains and discusses this with her in more detail.

Unfortunately, the evidence of tests and observation establish that Mrs Green has poor bladder function, and in view of her general disability, she is advised to have a permanent urethral catheter in order to improve her quality of life. (Now refer to the Nursing Care Plan for Mrs Green.)

Potential entry sites for infection in closed-circuit urinary drainage

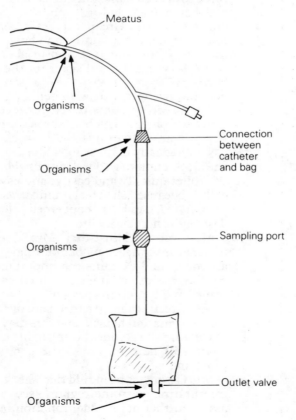

Meatus

Organisms

Connection between catheter and bag

Organisms

Sampling port

Organisms

Outlet valve

Organisms

Nursing Care Plan for Mrs Green

PROBLEM	NATURE	NURSING ACTION AND RATIONALE	EVALUATION
Actual	Mrs Green is anxious at the prospect of being catheterised.	Margaret spends time with Mrs Green discussing her anxieties, and is then able to reassure her. She explains how the catheter is inserted and how it is retained by the balloon. She reassures Mrs Green that it will cause minimal discomfort, and that it will relieve her current problems and enable her to enjoy her life more than at present. By explaining the procedure she hopes to relieve some of Mrs Green's anxiety.	Although Mrs Green had been prepared for the possibility of a catheter, she had not asked any questions about the procedure involved, as she had suppressed the idea in her thoughts. Margaret's reassuring explanations helped her to accept the situation more easily.
Actual	Mrs Green is very distressed about the prospects of a permanent catheter.	Margaret listens to Mrs Green's fears. It is important that she has the opportunity to express her concern about the effect of a catheter on her self-concept and body image. Margaret encourages her to discuss her fears with her husband, and suggests that they talk together to the doctor, even though they may feel embarrassed.	After discussion with the doctor and also with the Ward Sister, Mrs Green feels better able to accept her catheter. Her husband offers a great deal of support. She is particularly relieved to know that the presence of the catheter will not prevent a continuing sexual relationship between them.

Nursing Care Plan for Mrs Green

PROBLEM	NATURE	NURSING ACTION AND RATIONALE	EVALUATION
Potential	Urinary tract infection due to the presence of a urethral catheter.	Margaret explains to Mrs Green the points where infection can enter the drainage system. She discusses with her the importance of cleaning the urethral meatus with soap and water at least twice per day, and other potential entry sites for micro-organisms with an appropriate agent (e.g. 70% methylated spirit). She encourages her to maintain a fluid intake of 2–3 litres in each 24 hours to avoid stasis of urine which enables rapid colonisation by micro-organisms. Margaret also advises her that the tubing and collection bag should remain below the level of the bladder to prevent retrograde flow of urine.	Mrs Green cares for her catheter well, maintaining the required fluid intake, and cleaning the drainage system in the correct way. As a result, she remains free of infection.

Prior to Mrs Green returning home, Margaret shows her how to empty her collection bags and how to change them. She also provides Mrs Green with supervised practice to ensure that she can cope with these tasks.

The use of leg-fastening drainage bags is discussed, and Mrs Green commences use of these during the day before going home. She finds these more suitable as they can be disguised beneath a skirt or trousers. She changes to the use of large bags at night.

Mrs Green is given a sheet of paper on which all the information for dealing with the catheter is listed for her easy referral as necessary. Her husband is also involved in the preparation for going home, so that, should she be unwell, he is able to deal with the catheter for her. She is very much looking forward to being home with her family.

Summary of advice given to Mrs Green

1 Catheter toilet should be performed twice per day and after bowel action to avoid contamination.
2 Drink 2–3 litres per 24 hours.
3 Always wash your hands thoroughly before and after dealing with the catheter and changing bags.
4 Each bag should be washed in mild detergent after use and hung to dry. Bags should be changed weekly.
5 Ensure free drainage by avoiding kinked tubing and keeping the bag below bladder level. Avoid constipation as this can prevent proper drainage.
6 If you have any queries about the drainage or the catheter contact your District Nurse. If you are in discomfort or pain and no urine drains, *seek immediate help* (e.g. your GP).

Urinary retention is when a patient is unable to pass urine at all, and the bladder becomes painfully distended.

Nursing Mr Robertson who requires a supra-pubic catheter

Mr James Robertson is a 68-year-old retired factory foreman who lives alone. He is a widower, his wife having died 10 years previously. Since her death he has occupied himself in his retirement with his garden and allotment. He takes great pride in his flowers and vegetables with which he often wins prizes at local shows. He shares the produce with his friends at the local pub where he plays darts several evenings per week.

During the past year, he has experienced difficulties with micturition, having to go to the toilet more frequently. His friends at the pub had observed this, and one suggested he should visit his GP.

He is, however, rather embarrassed, and manages to cope until one afternoon he is unable to pass urine at all and is in considerable discomfort. He is admitted to the ward via the Accident and Emergency Department, having been diagnosed as having urinary retention.

On arrival in the ward, Mr Robertson is welcomed by Margaret, the ward nurse, who has a bed ready for him. She settles him into bed and unpacks the few belongings he has with him. He is rather distressed at being admitted, and the extreme discomfort he experienced has made him rather anxious and frightened.

His main discomfort has been relieved by the insertion of a supra-pubic catheter in the Accident and Emergency Department. This was carried out under local anaesthetic as it was not possible to pass a urethral catheter because of apparent obstruction.

Owing to the large volume of urine in Mr

The position of a supra-pubic catheter

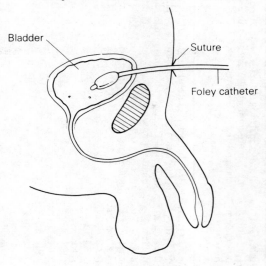

Bladder

Suture

Foley catheter

Robertson's bladder, the catheter tubing was clamped after initial drainage of 500–1000 ml. (This practice may vary according to surgeons' preference.)

Margaret then releases the clamp at intervals over a period of time. (This prevents the possible complications of sudden bladder decompression, for example, shock, or reactionary haemorrhage from the capillary network of the bladder wall.) She records all urine output on a fluid-balance chart. (Refer now to the Nursing Care Plan for Mr Robertson.)

FURTHER CARE

Mr Robertson's condition is now stable. He will remain in hospital with the supra-pubic catheter *in situ* while investigations are carried out to confirm the provisional diagnosis. He will then most probably have surgery to his prostate gland – a *prostatectomy* (see Chapter 7).

Nursing Care Plan for Mr Robertson

PROBLEM	NATURE	NURSING CARE AND RATIONALE	EVALUATION
Actual	Abdominal pain and discomfort following urinary retention and insertion of a supra-pubic catheter.	Margaret ensures that Mr Robertson is given adequate analgesia as prescribed. He is already anxious, and his concern will only be exacerbated if he is not comfortable.	Effective analgesia makes Mr Robertson much more comfortable, and he is able to relax and discuss his anxieties.
Actual	Anxiety about the possible cause of the retention.	Margaret discusses with Mr Robertson the information given to him by the doctor who treated him in the Accident and Emergency Department. He was informed that he probably has an enlarged prostate gland. She reinforces this explanation by reassuring him that this is a common problem for a gentleman in his age group, and his history would seem to point to this problem. She draws a simple diagram to aid his understanding and explains that he will require investigations to confirm the diagnosis. Although he has been given information by the doctor, his stress was such at the time that he was unable to absorb it all, and this further discussion was therefore necessary.	Mr Robertson is grateful for Margaret's information, and feels reassured about his situation. The doctor had told him he might require an operation, and he is able to accept this with his improved understanding of the situation.

Potential	Urinary tract infection due to the presence of a catheter.	The supra-pubic catheter entering the bladder via the abdominal wall provides ideal access for micro-organisms. Margaret ensures, therefore, that the site is clean and dry where the catheter is sutured to the abdominal wall, and that it is protected by a sterile dressing. She observes for signs of infection, i.e. redness, swelling or discharge at the site, and monitors his temperature every four hours. She also ensures correct care of the drainage system, and encourages a fluid intake of 2–3 litres per 24 hours.	Mr Robertson's catheter drains well, and he remains free of infection.

(Now turn back to p. 25).

27

The prostate gland. (a) The normal position of the
prostate gland. (b) An enlarged prostate gland, showing its
effects

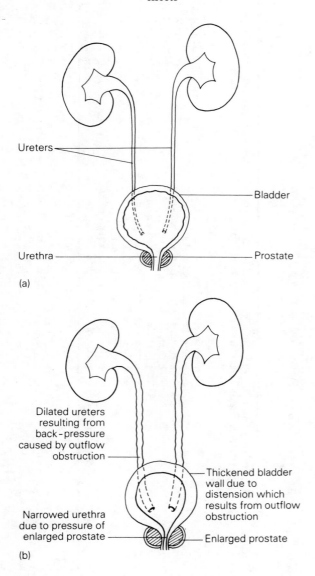

Ureters

Bladder

Urethra

Prostate

(a)

Dilated ureters
resulting from
back-pressure
caused by outflow
obstruction

Thickened bladder
wall due to
distension which
results from outflow
obstruction

Narrowed urethra
due to pressure of
enlarged prostate

Enlarged prostate

(b)

Further information about catheters

The two patients whose care has been discussed in this chapter both required catheterisation. As stated in Chapter 1, many patients on this ward will require catheters for a variety of reasons, and it is important for you to understand some significant points relating to their use.

You now need to know the rationale behind the selection of different types and sizes of catheter. On occasions such as surgery, the doctor selects the catheter to be used, but in the ward the nursing staff will be involved in the decision as they often perform the procedure. The following information may be helpful to you regarding the selection of catheters.

TYPES OF CATHETER

Type of catheter may refer to the style of catheter or to the material from which it is made.

Style
Catheters may differ in length, the number of outlet holes at the tip, and the number of channels within the catheter.

As the female urethra is much shorter than the male, two lengths of catheter are manufactured. The outlet holes at the tip vary in number, position and size. The Roberts catheter, for example, has one outlet hole below the balloon to facilitate drainage.

The number of channels within the lumen may vary. Two-way catheters have one channel for urine drainage, and one for inflation and deflation of the balloon. Three-way catheters have an additional channel which allows for fluid to enter the bladder, e.g. irrigation following surgery.

Types of material

Latex Rubber Catheters
These are suitable for short term use only, i.e. up to 10 days. The latex can be irritant to the urethral mucosa, and prolonged use may lead to the development of cracks and encrustations. These catheters are relatively cheap.

Coated-Latex Catheters
The coating may be PVC Silicone or Teflon. These are suitable for medium-term use (4–6 weeks). They tend to have a narrower lumen because of the coating, which does however reduce the incidence of chemical urethritis.

Silicone Catheters
These are made from 100% silicone. The internal lumen, therefore, tends to be larger. The silicone is said to be physiologically inert, thus causing minimal urethral irritation. Such catheters are the most expensive, but are suitable for long-term use – approximately 3 months.

Many claims are made about materials used in catheter manufacture; the above information, however, should provide broad guidelines, bearing in mind that each patient is an individual with an individual problem.

SIZE OF CATHETER

The size of catheter is measured on the Charrière (Ch.) or French Gauge (f.g.). The terms are synonymous and represent the external circumference of the catheter in millimetres by 2-mm steps.

Sizes 12–16 are suitable for most adults requiring standard drainage.

BALLOON SIZE

Each catheter is marked with the maximum amount of water to be used to inflate the balloon: 5 ml is adequate for most patients. It ensures the minimum residual urine beneath the balloon, minimum pressure on the bladder neck, and reduces irritation of the bladder which results in contractions or 'bladder spasm' and subsequent leakage.

The golden rule when selecting the size of catheter is to choose the smallest catheter and smallest size of balloon for the required purpose.

TEST YOURSELF

1 What are the indications for inserting a urinary catheter?
2 Why did Mrs Green require a catheter?
3 What advice did Mrs Green receive about catheter hygiene?
4 What information was given to Mrs Green on her return home?
5 What was the possible cause of Mr Robertson's urinary retention?
6 Why did Mr Robertson have a supra-pubic rather than a urethral catheter?
7 Which type of catheter was most suitable for Mr Robertson's problem?
8 Which rules are applied when selecting a catheter?

FURTHER READING

Blannin, J. P. 1982. Catheter management. *Nursing Times*, 17th March 1982, 438–440.
Conference Proceedings. 1982. *Urinary Tract Infection: The Role of the Nurse*. Nursing Practice Research Unit. Northwick Park Hospital, Harrow, Middlesex.
Jenner, E. A. *et al.* 1983. Catheterization and urinary tract infection. *Nursing* (2nd series), No. 3, supplement May 1983, 1–7. London: Medical Education.
Royal Marsden Hospital 1984. *Manual of Clinical Policies and Procedures*. Lippincott Nursing series. London: Harper and Row.
Seth, C. 1986. Which catheter? *Nursing Times*, supplement on Community Outlook, September 1986.

4 Caring for a patient who has haematuria

HISTORY

Mrs Joan Wallace is a 50-year-old lady who is married and has a grown-up family. She runs her own hairdressing business, and one of her three daughters helps her with this. Her husband's job involves a considerable amount of travelling, and he is often away for several weeks at a time.

On a number of occasions during the past four weeks Mrs Wallace has noticed the presence of blood when passing urine. She was unsure initially where the blood was coming from. She had reached the menopause three years previously and had since suffered no vaginal blood loss, which led her to conclude that the blood was coming from her urinary system.

She had experienced cystitis (inflammation of the bladder) on two occasions in the past, and had noted the presence of blood then. On those occasions, however, there was extreme discomfort on passing urine, together with frequency and urgency, whereas now the haematuria was painless. Following the third episode of haematuria she visited her GP who referred her to the urological clinic. As a result the following week she was admitted for investigation to establish the cause of the problem.

Haematuria is the presence of blood in the urine.

Haematuria is caused by:
1 Urinary calculi (stones).
2 Infection or inflammation, of the urinary tract.
3 Trauma to the urinary system.
4 Malignant disease of the urinary tract.

<table>
<tr><td>

INITIAL
NURSING
CARE

</td></tr>
</table>

On arrival in the ward, Mrs Wallace appears very anxious. Margaret, the ward nurse, shows her to her bed and explains the ward facilities to her.

Mrs Wallace is very concerned about being admitted, as she thought her problem to be quite minor, and is worried about her business while she is in hospital. Her husband is away from home on business at present.

Margaret reassures her that her stay will not be lengthy – probably no longer than a week – and that the investigations will be carried out as quickly as possible. The doctor has informed Mrs Wallace about the tests required, and Margaret is able to discuss these with her again, as she found it difficult to take in all the details at the time of the clinic visit.

Margaret explains initial tests which will be carried out on the ward. These tests are:

1 Routine Urinalysis
This is testing a freshly voided sample with a reagent strip. Margaret would expect to find blood and protein due to the presence of red blood cells in the urine.

2 MSU
MSU is the collection of a midstream specimen of urine. This would be a specimen as free from outside contamination as possible, obtained by cleansing the vulval area, then asking the patient to pass urine into the toilet, then stop; then pass some urine into a sterile container before finishing into the toilet. The specimen is sent to the Microbiology Department for culture and antibiotic sensitivity

testing. This will reveal any infection and any abnormal cells present.

3 Full Blood Count
This includes full analysis of a blood sample, including estimation of haemoglobin, which will indicate if Mrs Wallace is anaemic as a result of blood loss. It will also provide details of the white blood cell count, indicating infection if this is raised.

Margaret also clarifies with Mrs Wallace the preparation for the X-ray of her urinary system – an *intravenous urogram* (IVU). Mrs Wallace is grateful for the information given to her about the investigations, and is less anxious.

An intravenous urogram is an X-ray investigation using radio-opaque dye to obtain a picture of the urinary system. Preparation is important in order that clear pictures can be obtained. If the bowel is loaded with faeces this will obstruct the view. Laxatives are therefore prescribed the night prior to the IVU. Food is withheld 4 hours before and fluids 2 hours before the test. Fluids are withheld to enable better concentration of the dye, and thus clearer pictures. (There are variations in local policy for preparation, but the principles are the same.) The patient has a bath, and puts on a gown. The procedure is not painful, but may be uncomfortable while X-ray pictures are taken over a period of approximately 30 minutes.

Cystoscopy involves examination of the inside of the bladder under local epidural or general anaesthetic. A fibre-optic instrument called a *cystoscope*, passed through the urethra, enables examination of the bladder, and biopsy of tissue if necessary.

The intravenous urogram result shows that the dye has not filled the bladder in a uniform way. (There is what is termed 'a filling defect'.)

The doctor explains to Mrs Wallace that, in order to examine her bladder further, they would like to perform a *cystoscopy*. Four days after admission Mrs Wallace goes to theatre for a cystoscopy under general anaesthetic. Margaret has explained that she will feel some discomfort initially when passing urine post-operatively, and that the procedure is a very minor one.

A cystoscope

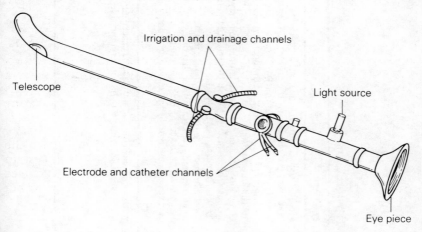

Telescope

Irrigation and drainage channels

Light source

Electrode and catheter channels

Eye piece

The cystoscopy reveals two small tumours of the bladder. They are treated with *diathermy*, and a biopsy is sent to the laboratory for analysis as these are thought to be malignant. Mrs Wallace returns to the ward and recovers quickly from the anaesthetic.

Diathermy of bladder tumours Using the cystoscope, an electrode is manipulated into contact with the tumour. A diathermy (or current of high frequency) is discharged into it, thus burning and destroying it.

The following morning the doctor visits her and explains what was found at the operation. Margaret is present when he talks with her, so that she is aware of what has been said. Mrs Wallace is told that her two small tumours are probably malignant, but that they must wait for confirmation. She is also told that they have been completely removed, and that she can look positively to the future as she may well not have any recurrence. (Refer now to the Post-operative Nursing Care Plan for Mrs Wallace.)

Post-operative Nursing Care Plan for Mrs Wallace

ACTUAL PROBLEM	NURSING CARE AND RATIONALE	EVALUATION
Anxiety about her diagnosis.	Margaret encourages Mrs Wallace to express her concerns, and gives her the opportunity to talk at length while awaiting the biopsy result.	Mrs Wallace remains anxious, but appreciates the opportunity to discuss the problems. The histology report confirms that Mrs Wallace has carcinoma of the bladder, and the doctor gives her this information. Her husband has now arrived home, and they are both able to discuss the matter with the doctor. He reassures Mrs Wallace that she will require frequent cystoscopies to monitor her condition, and is able to tell her that many patients are still coming for these 'check cystoscopies' after 10–15 years and are fit and well.
Post-operative haematuria and urethral discomfort on passing urine.	Margaret had prepared Mrs Wallace to expect this, and she advises her to drink 2–3 litres of fluid per 24 hours for 2–3 days until the urine becomes clear. The increased fluids 'flush through' the urinary system. Analgesia is also given as prescribed for the discomfort.	Within two days the haematuria has ceased and Mrs Wallace is feeling much more comfortable.

Mrs Wallace is feeling much better at the end of the week. She has had ample opportunity to discuss her condition with her husband and the doctor. She is eager to return home and get back to her business.

Before she leaves hospital for home, Margaret explains once more the importance of regular check cystoscopies. She will initially come every three months, but if she is well and no recurrence of tumour is seen, the intervals will extend to six months and, eventually, yearly. She will not need to be in hospital for more than an overnight stay, and this should not disrupt her business too much, for which she is very grateful.

Margaret also reminds her that if she has any haematuria or symptoms of urinary infection, she should visit her GP without delay to ensure prompt treatment, as these symptoms may indicate some recurrence of tumour. Prompt treatment is emphasised as important to ensure the condition does not become more serious.

Mrs Wallace is less anxious and distressed now that she has a good understanding of her condition. She is relieved that she can return to work, and she and her husband plan a short holiday prior to her next admission.

1 What was the cause of Mrs Wallace's haematuria?
2 Prior to Mrs Wallace having an intravenous urogram, what were the nurse's responsibilities?
3 Why did Mrs Wallace require diathermy via the cystoscope?
4 What significant information did Mrs Wallace require on returning home?

FURTHER READING

Blandy, J. 1982. *Lecture Notes on Urology*. 3rd Ed. Oxford: Blackwell Scientific Publications.

Charlton, C. A. C. 1984. *The Urological System*. 2nd Ed. London: Churchill Livingstone.

Wallis, M. C. 1984. The collection and testing of urine. *Nursing* (2nd series), No. 29, September 1984, 853–855.

5 Caring for a patient who has urinary colic

HISTORY

Mr Peter Hunt is a 40-year-old painter and decorator who works for a large building firm. He is married with three children, and his wife has a part-time job as a school secretary.

One morning soon after starting work, Mr Hunt began to experience pain in his side. Initially, he ignored this, but after two hours the bouts of pain became very severe. He had to stop work, and one of the colleagues with whom he worked brought him to the hospital.

On arrival in the Accident and Emergency Department he described the pain as passing in waves from his right loin to his right groin. It was very severe and made him feel nauseous. Mr Hunt was examined by the doctor who diagnosed urinary colic and decided to admit him to the ward for investigation and treatment. He also prescribed a strong intramuscular analgesic to alleviate his pain. The Accident and Emergency Department nurse contacted his wife and his employer to inform them of his admission.

Urinary colic is characterised by waves of severe pain, resulting from powerful contraction of the smooth muscle in the renal pelvis or ureter. It is usually caused by the presence of a calculus, or stone, which is obstructing the urinary flow. The calculus may form because urine can be predisposed to precipitation of its constituents.

INITIAL NURSING CARE

On arrival in the ward, Mr Hunt is feeling exhausted and generally unwell. Margaret, the ward nurse, makes him comfortable in bed in his preferred position so that he can rest. His pain has been relieved by the injection, and a full nursing history obtained when he has had some rest.

Predisposing factors to the formation of urinary calculi
1   Immobility.
2   Disorders of metabolism.
3   Foreign bodies in the urinary tract.
4   Dehydration.
5   Obstruction of the urinary tract causing urinary stasis.

After three hours' rest and some sleep, Mr Hunt is feeling better and is still pain-free. Margaret assists him to have a wash as he has been perspiring a great deal, and soon he feels more comfortable.

He is very concerned, however, about his possible length of stay in hospital. With three children, he cannot afford to be away from work, as he is dependent upon overtime to boost his income.

Margaret explains that he may pass the calculus spontaneously and require no further treatment, but that if not, it is in his own long-term interest to have the problem investigated and treated as appropriate. Investigation may help to reveal the cause of the stone.

Margaret asks Mr Hunt to pass all his urine into a urinal, even if using the toilet, in order that it can be sieved for the presence of calculi. She also records fluid intake and output on a fluid balance chart. (Now refer to the Nursing Care Plan for Mr Hunt.)

Nursing Care Plan for Mr Hunt

PROBLEM	NATURE	NURSING CARE AND RATIONALE	EVALUATION
Actual	Severe bouts of pain felt in waves from loin to groin, and sometimes at the tip of the penis and in the scrotum.	He is given prescribed analgesia regularly. (The drug used most commonly is Pethidine, which also has anti-spasmodic properties.) Margaret advises him to find the position most comfortable for him. This can be walking about (providing his analgesia does not make him unsteady), or lying in bed.	Mr Hunt's pain is controlled by the analgesia, and he spends most of his time in bed as this is most comfortable for him.
Actual	Nausea associated with severe pain.	Margaret ensures that Mr Hunt receives regular anti-emetic injections as prescribed with the analgesia. She provides him with a vomit bowl, tissues and a mouthwash in case he might vomit.	Mr Hunt does not vomit, and the anti-emetic does relieve his nausea.
Actual	Difficulty in eating and drinking due to pain and nausea.	Mr Hunt is encouraged to take food and fluids when nausea and pain subside. Margaret advises him that he should try to drink 2–3 litres of fluid per 24 hours; this helps to 'flush through' the urinary system, and encourage movement of the calculus.	Mr Hunt takes some food and fluids as able. He finds it difficult to achieve the fluid intake target because of his general condition, and, therefore, an intravenous infusion is commenced to ensure adequate hydration.

Nursing Care Plan for Mr Hunt

PROBLEM	NATURE	NURSING CARE AND RATIONALE	EVALUATION
Actual	Difficulty and discomfort when passing urine.	Margaret ensures that Mr Hunt has privacy to pass urine. She encourages him to stand up to pass urine, as this is a more natural position than lying in bed. Analgesia is given as prescribed to alleviate the discomfort.	As Mr Hunt's fluid intake increases with the infusion, his difficulty improves. He passes small amounts of tiny particles of calculus which account for the discomfort, but he still does not pass a calculus.
Potential	Urinary tract infection due to the presence of a calculus.	Margaret explains to Mr Hunt that the calculus will impair the urinary flow and stasis of urine may occur, which can result in infection. She therefore takes his temperature and pulse every four hours to monitor any increase which may indicate infection. She also collects a specimen of urine (MSU) for laboratory testing to look for infection (see Chapter 3).	Mr Hunt does not develop any infection. All observations are within normal limits, and the MSU does not culture any micro-organisms. This can be attributed to his good level of hydration.

Common sites for the formation of urinary calculi

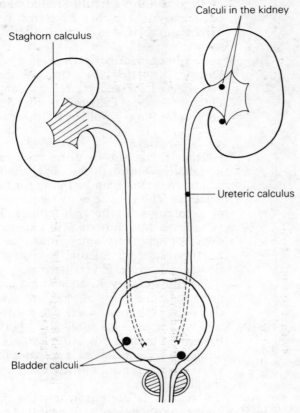

Staghorn calculus

Calculi in the kidney

Ureteric calculus

Bladder calculi

During the five days following his admission, Mr Hunt has several investigations aimed at establishing where the calculus is, and looking for a cause. These investigations were as follows:

1 Blood tests

These were for raised levels of calcium, uric acid, phosphate and cystine, as these are all well-known constituents of calculi. Increased serum quantities will result in an increased amount excreted in the urine which can precipitate to form calculi. Should abnormality be discovered, further investigation can be carried out related to the particular substance.

2 A 24-hour urine collection

During this period, the entire volume of urine is collected for analysis of its constituents. Once again, any abnormal results outside the acceptable range would be followed up.

3 IVU (see p. 34)

Neither the serum or urine tests reveal any metabolic abnormalities, and, therefore, no conclusive cause can be found for Mr Hunt's calculus. The IVU demonstrates the presence of a calculus in the right ureter. From the symptoms Mr Hunt is still experiencing, it does not appear to be moving. This is a very common site for a calculus to obstruct urinary flow, as the ureter is very narrow.

Mr Hunt is very anxious at his lack of progress, because of his absence from work, and the doctor suggests that the solution is to remove the calculus surgically – performing a *ureterolithotomy*. Mr Hunt is eager for the situation to be resolved, and, after discussing what the operation will involve, he agrees to the suggestion.

A ureterolithotomy involves an incision into the ureter to remove the calculus. It may be performed via a flank incision if the upper two-thirds of the ureter is affected, or abdominal for the lower one-third.

Margaret is present when the doctor explains the operation, and she follows this with more information about what to expect after the operation. She tells him that he will still have his intravenous infusion, he will have an incision covered by a dressing, and probably two drains from the wound site. She informs him that he will continue to receive analgesia for any discomfort.

Mr Hunt is then prepared for surgery in the routine manner, and returns to the ward via the recovery room. (Now refer to the Postoperative Nursing Care Plan for Mr Hunt.)

Post-operative Nursing Care Plan for Mr Hunt

PROBLEM	NATURE	NURSING CARE AND RATIONALE	EVALUATION
Potential	Haemorrhage following surgery.	Margaret observes the wound for excessive bleeding, and the wound drain to ensure it is not filling with an excessive quantity of blood. She monitors Mr Hunt's blood pressure and pulse which will indicate haemorrhage and the resulting reduction of circulatory volume. She also ensures that Mr Hunt remains well-hydrated, any fluid loss being replaced by monitoring his IVI.	Mr Hunt's dressing remains dry, and the wound drain contains only 30 ml of blood. His blood pressure and pulse remain within normal limits.
Actual	Reduced mobility due to surgery affects Mr Hunt's independence to carry out personal hygiene.	Margaret assists Mr Hunt to wash, allowing him as much independence as possible.	Mr Hunt is able to perform most activities independently, thus maintaining dignity.
Potential	Reduced activity may lead to venous stasis, and thence to deep vein thrombosis.	Margaret encourages Mr Hunt to carry out leg exercises, and sit out of bed for short periods from the first post-operative day.	Mr Hunt exercises well and takes short walks with help, thus maintaining adequate circulation.

Post-operative Nursing Care Plan for Mr Hunt

PROBLEM	NATURE	NURSING CARE AND RATIONALE	EVALUATION
Actual	Pain from the incision, and difficulty in taking deep breaths due to the flank wound directly below the diaphragm.	Margaret ensures that Mr Hunt has adequate analgesia to allow him maximum respiratory movement. The physiotherapist discusses the importance of deep breathing to prevent chest infection, and Margaret encourages Mr Hunt to breathe deeply regularly.	With adequate analgesia and encouragement Mr Hunt is able to manage deep breathing exercises and avoids chest infection.
Potential	Dehydration due to blood loss at surgery and reduced oral fluid intake immediately post-operatively.	Mr Hunt is encouraged to drink small amounts of fluid as soon as he feels able, building up to free fluids. Oral fluids are introduced gradually to prevent abdominal distension (or paralytic ileus) which can develop because the bowel and kidney have common innervation. In the meantime Margaret ensures that his IVI runs at the correct rate to maintain hydration. She observes the site of the infusion to ensure it is not inflamed, which could jeopardise the infusion.	Mr Hunt remains well-hydrated with the infusion, and does not develop abdominal distension. By the third post-operative day he is drinking and eating, and the infusion is discontinued.

| Potential | Impaired urine output from right kidney, due to oedema of the ureter following surgery. | Margaret ensures that Mr Hunt's urine output is accurately measured and recorded on the fluid balance chart along with fluid intake. She records separately the output via a T-Tube drain, inserted in the right ureter so that renal function on both sides can be monitored. (A **T-Tube** is a fine tube drain inserted in the ureter following surgery. It ensures drainage of urine from the kidney on the operated side, maintaining patency of the ureter. It also acts to prevent leakage of urine, as the ureter is not sutured in order to avoid later stricture from scarring.) | Mr Hunt maintains adequate volumes of output, both via the urethral catheter and the T-Tube. The T-Tube drainage diminishes after two days, and on the third day it is removed. The urethral catheter is also removed, and Mr Hunt passes urine urethrally without difficulty. |
| Potential | Infection of wound and drain sites. | Aseptic technique is used by Margaret whenever she cares for the incision line or the drainage tubes, thus avoiding contamination. She observes for signs of inflammation, swelling, redness or discharge which would indicate the presence of infection, and monitors Mr Hunt's temperature every four hours for the same reason. | Mr Hunt's wound heals well. His wound drain is removed after four days, and his sutures after 10 days. (The T-Tube was removed on day 3.) |

Mr Hunt returns home after more than two weeks in hospital. He is very relieved that his calculus has been removed, although, unfortunately (as with a majority of patients with urinary calculi) no cause was found for his problem.

His wife and children are looking forward to having him back home after his absence. He is very keen to return to work, but Margaret explains to him that he should not return to his job until seen in the Outpatient Clinic after one month. He has had a large operation, and the tissues need to be fully healed before he starts painting and decorating which involves climbing and stretching. Fortunately, Mr Hunt's employer has been very understanding, and this alleviates much of his anxiety about work.

Lithotripsy

This is a new non-invasive technique for disintegrating kidney stones, and was first introduced to the United Kingdom in 1984. The sound of energy waves can be focused to concentrate on a kidney stone (whilst not harming the tissues) until it breaks into sand-like particles which can be flushed away in the urinary stream.

The treatment is performed under general or epidural anaesthetic, and involves the patient being partially immersed in a bath of water which is used to transmit the pressure waves to the calculus.

As this is non-invasive, it reduces the length of stay in hospital, and minimises potential complications of major surgery.

TEST
YOURSELF

1   What were the predisposing factors for the formation of urinary calculi?

2   What was Mr Hunt's most important problem on admission, and how was it resolved?
3   What were the significant points of Mr Hunt's nursing care in relation to fluid intake and output?
4   Why was Mr Hunt's calculus removed by surgical means?
5   Why did Mr Hunt require a T-tube drain post-operatively?
6   Why might Mr Hunt have had difficulty with breathing post-operatively?

FURTHER READING

Davidson, R. & McVey, P. 1985. Extra-corporeal shock wave lithotripsy. *Nursing Times*, September 11th 1985, 24–27.
Hayward, J. 1975. *Information: A Prescription Against Pain*. London: RCN.
Winter, C. C. & Movel, A. 1977. *Nursing Care of Patients with Urological Diseases*. 4th Ed. St. Louis: The C. V. Mosby Co.

6 Caring for a patient who is undergoing a nephrectomy

(see p. 34)

HISTORY

A **staghorn calculus** often develops through infection of the urine. It grows to fill the renal pelvis and calices – in the shape of a stag's horns. The calculus obstructs the flow of urine. In time, it causes renal damage and greatly reduces renal function.

Miss Mary Westgate is a 45-year-old lady living with her elderly mother who has severe arthritis, and who is quite dependent upon her daughter. Miss Westgate works as personal secretary to the director of a local company, which is a job she very much enjoys. Over the past two years she has had several episodes of cystitis and generalised urinary tract infection. These have been not only uncomfortable and unpleasant, but have made her feel embarrassed at work, making frequent trips to the toilet.

On the most recent occasion she felt very unwell indeed, and was away from work for a week. She experienced not only dysuria (difficult and painful micturition), but also haematuria, back ache, nausea and high temperatures.

Her GP had treated the infection with antibiotics, but when she had recovered he felt that she should have further investigation of this long-running problem. She had an IVU (see p. 34) as an outpatient, which demonstrated a large staghorn calculus in the pelvis of the left kidney.

Miss Westgate is referred to the Outpatient Clinic, and the doctor informs her that the

A staghorn calculus

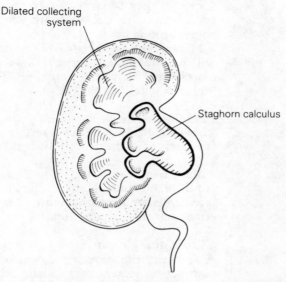

Dilated collecting system

Staghorn calculus

calculus will have to be removed. Prior to this, investigation of her urinary system is necessary. He explains that if the kidney damage is severe, removal of the kidney (nephrectomy) may be necessary, although this is not always the case. Miss Westgate arranges for a relative to come and care for her mother, and is then admitted to hospital.

INITIAL NURSING CARE

On admission to the ward Miss Westgate is welcomed by Margaret, the ward nurse. She is very anxious, both about leaving a relative to care for her mother (as she is unfamiliar with her mother's routine), and about the possibility of losing her left kidney.

Although she had some discussion with the doctor in the clinic, Margaret encourages her to express her anxieties, and talks through the problem with her. She suggests that Miss

Westgate writes down any questions for the doctor as they occur to her, in order that she doesn't omit to ask anything when next he comes around.

Margaret explains to Miss Westgate that she will require some routine urological tests to assess the extent of her problem. These tests include the following:

1 MSU
This establishes whether there is still infection present in the urinary system.

2 Blood tests
A full blood count is made; urea and electrolyte levels are noted, which will indicate the efficiency of renal function.

3 Creatinine clearance
A 24-hour urine-save is performed, which on completion is sent to the laboratory with a venous blood sample. Analysis of both reveal the rate at which creatinine is cleared by the kidney, (i.e. the glomerular filtration rate).

The IVU which Miss Westgate underwent as an outpatient revealed a very extensive calculus, and the remaining investigations confirm that it has caused sufficient damage for the renal function to be seriously impaired. The doctor informs Miss Westgate that nephrectomy is advisable.

Although Miss Westgate was in some way prepared for the news, Margaret spends long periods of time discussing the operation with her. She has few friends, being committed to looking after her mother, and feels she has no-one with whom to discuss her problems. She is anxious about the operation itself, and about the prospect of having only one kidney.

Margaret arranges for the ward sister and doctor to talk this over with Miss Westgate, and she is present so that she can hear the information given. Miss Westgate is assured that her life need be no different with one kidney. She will be able to continue her job, and to continue to care for her mother.

Margaret explains to Miss Westgate what she may expect post-operatively. She assures her that she will have analgesia for pain, and that she will have a flank wound and a wound drain. She will also have an IVI. From four hours before her operation she will have nothing to eat or drink to reduce the risk of inhaling vomit under anaesthetic (Hamilton-Smith 1972).

On the day of the operation Margaret makes Miss Westgate's bed with clean linen, while she bathes and puts on an operation gown. Miss Westgate removes all jewellery, make-up, and her dentures.

Margaret ensures that she has an identity band on, and that her consent form is signed. She advises Miss Westgate to pass urine before getting into bed and receiving her pre-medication which, Margaret explains, will make her sleepy and her mouth dry.

Margaret accompanied Miss Westgate to theatre, and this, together with the detailed discussion and preparation for the operation, helped her to feel less anxious. (Now refer to the Post-operative Nursing Care Plan for Miss Westgate.)

RETURNING HOME

Miss Westgate is ready to return home after two weeks. She has made an uneventful post-operative recovery. She is concerned about restrictions on her future lifestyle with only one kidney. Margaret arranges for her to see the doctor again, and is present at the discussion.

The doctor emphasises that she need not alter her lifestyle in any way. If she wishes, and

Post-operative Nursing Care Plan for Miss Westgate

PROBLEM	NATURE	NURSING CARE AND RATIONALE	EVALUATION
Potential	Haemorrhage following surgery.	Margaret observes the wound site for excessive bleeding. There is one wound drain, the drainage from which she monitors and records on the fluid-balance chart. Haemorrhage may manifest itself firstly by increased blood in the drainage bag and bleeding through the wound dressing. She also monitors Miss Westgate's pulse and blood pressure for increased pulse and decreased blood pressure – a sign of reduced circulatory volume caused by haemorrhage.	There is no sign of excessive bleeding from the wound or at the wound drain. Miss Westgate's observations remain stable.
Actual	Discomfort over incision on left flank.	Margaret ensures that analgesia is given regularly as prescribed. She finds positions in which Miss Westgate is most comfortable, and helps to position her, supported with pillows.	Miss Westgate's pain is well controlled, and she feels comfortable.
Potential	Chest infection due to flank incision inhibiting deep breathing.	Together with the physiotherapist, Margaret encourages Miss Westgate to carry out breathing exercises, after adequate analgesia to relieve the discomfort. The deep breathing encourages full lung expansion, and minimises the possibility of infection.	Miss Westgate carries out her exercises as instructed and avoids chest infection.

Potential	Dehydration due to reduced oral intake and fluid loss at surgery.	Miss Westgate is encouraged to drink as soon as she is fully awake, building up to free fluids. This will ensure hydration and encourage a good urine output. She has an IVI in the meantime which Margaret monitors, ensuring it runs at the correct rate.	Miss Westgate remains well-hydrated, and soon begins to drink freely. Her IVI is discontinued after two days. Her urine output is in balance with her intake, indicating sound function of her remaining kidney.
Potential	Wound infection, in particular, as Miss Westgate has had frequent infections.	Margaret observes the wound for discomfort, redness, swelling or discharge which would indicate infection. She also observes the drain site similarly. Aseptic technique is used at all times when caring for the wound and drain to prevent contamination. Margaret monitors Miss Westgate's temperature and pulse, as, if there is infection, these will be raised.	Miss Westgate's incision remains free of infection. The drain is removed after three days when drainage is minimal. The sutures are removed after 10 days.

in case of being involved in an accident, she may carry a card or some similar form of identification stating that she has only one kidney.

Miss Westgate is advised not to return to work before she has had her appointment in the Outpatient Clinic after one month. She should not try to hasten her recovery while tissues heal and she regains her strength. The doctor also advises her against doing too much for her mother as this time. Fortunately, the relative who has been helping is able to remain for several more weeks, so that Miss Westgate can have some rest. She is very relieved at the outcome of her operation, and appears to have accepted the situation well. She is looking forward to returning to work without her previous anxieties caused by persistent urine infections.

TEST YOURSELF

1 Which problem first caused Miss Westgate to visit her GP?
2 Why did Miss Westgate require a nephrectomy?
3 How did Miss Westgate feel about having a nephrectomy?
4 How could the nurses ensure that she had adequate information about her future?
5 What support was arranged for Miss Westgate at home?

FURTHER READING

Blandy, J. 1982. *Lecture Notes on Urology*. 3rd Ed. Oxford: Blackwell Scientific Publications.
Hamilton-Smith, S. 1972. *Nil by Mouth? A Descriptive Study of Nursing Care in Relation to Pre-operative Fasting*. London: RCN.

7 Caring for a patient who is undergoing prostatectomy

HISTORY

Mr Charles Webb is a 70-year-old gentleman who is married and lives with his wife in warden-assisted sheltered housing. His wife is severely disabled with arthritis, and relies on her husband to shop, cook and do some of the household chores. They have one daughter who lives in Australia, and whom they have not seen for several years, although she has invited them for a long holiday to see their two grandchildren.

Mr Webb has experienced urinary problems for approximately one year. His GP has attributed his symptoms to an enlarged prostate gland (see p. 28). (You will recall from Chapter 3 that this was the cause of Mr Robertson's urinary retention.) Mr Webb also has chronic bronchitis which troubles him mostly in the winter months, and as a result of which he gave up smoking five years ago.

Prostatism

What are the symptoms of prostatism?

1 Hesitancy
This occurs when the patient has a desire to pass urine, but experiences delay in actual voiding.

2 Dysuria
This is the term used to describe painful, difficult micturition.

3 Poor Stream
This means the urinary stream is much less powerful than previously.

4 Frequency
Here the patient requires to empty his bladder more frequently than before.

5 Dribbling Incontinence
This occurs due to residual urine in the bladder, not voided due to obstruction, which then leaks out when intra-abdominal pressure is increased.

6 Retention
This is the end result if prostatism is untreated, i.e. inability to void (see Chapter 3.)

Mr Webb has experienced most of these symptoms, but has never been in urinary retention. He has had investigations carried out as an outpatient, and the IVU (see p. 34) confirms that the prostate gland is enlarged. It also demonstrates dilatation of both ureters caused by back-pressure on the urinary flow from the obstruction.

Why does prostatic enlargement occur?
The true cause is unknown, although it is associated with advancing age, and, perhaps, disturbed testicular hormone production: 35% of men over 45 years have enlargement or hypertrophy of the prostate in varying degrees. Approximately 10% of patients with enlarged prostate glands have malignant disease or carcinoma of the prostate. In both instances, urinary symptoms have to be relieved by surgery, although the particular operation will depend on the precise diagnosis.

As a result, Mr Webb is admitted for surgery as prolonged back-pressure in the urinary system can cause renal damage, and therefore needs to be treated.

Prostatectomy is performed to remove prostatic tissue. *Retropubic prostatectomy* involves an abdominal incision through which the prostatic capsule is opened and the gland removed. *Trans-urethral resection of prostate* involves removing the prostatic tissue via the urethra, avoiding the abdominal incision and opening of the capsule.

Mr Webb is welcomed by Margaret, the ward nurse. He is very concerned about coming into hospital and leaving his wife, although he knows that the warden of their flats is going to call in on her very frequently, and has arranged for her to have a cooked meal every day. One or two neighbours who are quite fit have also agreed to visit. Margaret assures Mr Webb that anything he is concerned about at home can be dealt with, and that he need not worry, as the staff will do anything they can to help.

He is also concerned about his approaching surgery. He has never had an operation before, and is worried about his recovery and ability to continue caring for his wife.

Margaret spends a long time discussing Mr Webb's concerns with him. She makes every effort to give him the opportunity to talk through his anxieties. The approach of nurses to patients is a very important factor in allaying anxiety on admission to hospital (Franklin 1974). Mr Webb has been told that he will have a trans-urethral resection of prostate to improve his urinary problems.

Margaret is present when the doctor explains this to Mr Webb, and is then able to recap on some of the details. The doctor has also informed him that the anaesthetist will visit to examine his chest and assess his fitness for anaesthetic. It is decided by the doctors that Mr Webb should have his operation under epidural anaesthesia. They explain this to him, and Margaret follows this with more discussion to alleviate Mr Webb's anxieties. (Now refer to the Pre- and Post-operative Care Plans for Mr Webb.)

Pre-operative Nursing Care Plan for Mr Webb

ACTUAL PROBLEM	NURSING CARE AND RATIONALE	EVALUATION
Mr Webb is concerned about having an epidural anaesthetic.	Margaret reassures him that, although he will be conscious, the anaesthetist will ensure that he does not feel any pain, and that a nurse will be with him throughout the operation. She reinforces the doctor's explanation that he will make a quicker recovery, and so will have a shorter stay in hospital. She also reassures Mr Webb that any pain or discomfort he experiences after the operation can be easily controlled. Good explanation prior to surgery has been found to improve post-operative recovery and minimise pain (Hayward 1975).	Mr Webb is grateful for the time spent discussing and explaining the anaesthetic, and seems less anxious.
He is worried about the operation itself, and whether there will be complications.	Margaret assures him that he will be well prepared, and that the operation should be quite straightforward. So as not to alarm him after the operation, she tells him that he will have an intravenous infusion (IVI) *in situ* for 1–2 days because some local anaesthetics given via epidural cannula result in vasodilatation and, therefore, hypotension. The IVI could therefore be used to supplement his circulatory volume and maintain blood pressure. The intravenous infusion will also ensure adequate fluid intake and hydration throughout the operative period. He will also have a urethral	Mr Webb feels many of his fears are unfounded, and is less worried about his operation.

catheter and irrigation to wash through his bladder and prevent obstruction of the urinary flow by clots or debris from the operation. A collection of tubes entering and leaving the patient post-operatively are frightening if the patient is not prepared. Margaret explains that Mr Webb's urine will be blood-stained to start with. Again, this is alarming if the patient is unprepared. His observations will be recorded to monitor his progress. He is told that this is quite routine. He will also stay in bed for 12 hours, as the lower limbs are numbed, and he must wait for sensation to return. This is also routine.

Mr Webb is breathless on exertion.	Margaret ensures that he has sufficient pillows to sit up in bed in a comfortable position. He also has an armchair in which he can sit in an upright position, and thereby use his diaphragm to breathe more effectively. Margaret administers medication as prescribed to improve his respiratory function. She is also present when he is seen by the physiotherapist who teaches him some breathing exercises. In order that the pre-operative preparation is not too tiring, Margaret helps Mr Webb with a hoist bath, and assists him with the routine preparatory tasks to make him ready for theatre.	Mr Webb is ready for his operation in good time and without a rush, so that he is not breathless or over-anxious. He is appreciative of the assistance.

Post-operative Nursing Care Plan for Mr Webb

PROBLEM	NATURE	NURSING CARE AND RATIONALE	EVALUATION
Actual	Following epidural anaesthetic, Mr Webb must remain in bed for approximately 12 hours because of loss of sensation in the lower body.	Margaret makes Mr Webb comfortable, and explains again the need for 12 hours' bed rest. She maintains his observations, and assists him with a wash in bed when he feels ready.	Mr Webb makes a good post-operative recovery, and is up on the first day. He is pleased with his progress, and that he had an epidural anaesthetic.
Potential	Haemorrhage following surgery, as the prostate gland is a particularly vascular area, and haemostasis is more difficult to achieve using a trans-urethral approach.	Margaret observes the urine that is draining via the catheter, and notes the degree of haematuria. She also carries out observations of pulse and blood pressure to detect haemorrhage. A reduced circulatory volume will cause a raised pulse and lowered blood pressure.	Mr Webb has moderate haematuria for the first 24 hours, which becomes light on post-operative days 2 and 3. His observations remain stable.

Potential	Clot retention may occur. This is retention of urine in the bladder as a result of obstruction of the catheter by clots or fragments of clot.	Margaret ensures that Mr Webb's bladder irrigation is running accurately (see p. 67). He has intermittent irrigation in progress, and she ensures that the bags are replaced as prescribed, and that it is carried out with prescribed frequency so that no obstruction can occur from clots. She ensures that the contents of the urine-collection bag reflect the volume of irrigation instilled together with haematuria draining, and records this on the fluid-balance chart. She ensures that Mr Webb has no abdominal discomfort, as this may indicate increased volume in the bladder or clot retention.	Mr Webb's irrigation is carried out intermittently every half-hour immediately after his return from theatre, and then hourly after four hours. His catheter is draining moderate haematuria, and the irrigation is carried out every two hours during the night to ensure that he is not disturbed too frequently and gets some sleep. As light haematuria is draining by day 2, the irrigation is discontinued.
Potential	Dehydration due to reduced fluid intake over the operative period and fluid loss at operation.	Mr Webb's IVI is monitored by Margaret, ensuring the infusion rate is maintained, and observing the site for signs of inflammation. This ensures he stays adequately hydrated. Once able to drink on return to the ward, he is encouraged to drink 2–3 litres per 24 hours to ensure a good urine output which will flush the urinary system through and prevent urinary tract infection in the presence of the catheter.	The IVI is removed on the first post-operative day as Mr Webb is drinking well, and irrigation is still in progress.

Post-operative Nursing Care Plan for Mr Webb

PROBLEM	NATURE	NURSING CARE AND RATIONALE	EVALUATION
Actual	Restricted mobility due to Mr Webb having recently had an epidural, and having irrigation and catheter to cope with.	Mr Webb is assisted to mobilise when he is able to be up and about. He walks out to the washroom with assistance as he is rather breathless on exertion as before. He is assisted with personal hygiene by Margaret.	Mr Webb manages well with Margaret's help, and is pleased to regain some independence.
Actual	Embarrassment about Margaret helping him with catheter hygiene.	To minimise Mr Webb's embarrassment, Margaret shows him the importance of catheter toilet, and allows him privacy to perform this himself (see Chapter 3).	Mr Webb is able to carry out his own catheter hygiene, and feels less embarrassed. Twice weekly MSU reveals no infection present.
Potential	Catheter leakage due to bladder spasm, as result of the presence of the catheter balloon, and irrigation stimulating bladder contraction (see Chapter 3).	Margaret ensures that the irrigation, when running, is not over-filling Mr Webb's bladder. She also prepares him to expect some bladder spasm due to the catheter, and reminds him about catheter hygiene following leakage. She provides pads to place around the penis to protect his pyjamas.	Mr Webb has a minimal amount of leakage which he is able to deal with.

Potential	Constipation due to reduced mobility in the initial post-operative phase, and altered diet in hospital.	Mr Webb had not been constipated before the operation, but Margaret explains that worry and anxiety and altered diet in hospital can affect bowel function (Wright 1974). She therefore encourages Mr Webb to maintain a good fluid intake, as already discussed, and to eat foods with a high-fibre content. She explains that Mr Webb should avoid straining to achieve bowel action as it may induce haemorrhage due to the anatomical proximity of the rectum and prostate.	Unfortunately, Mr Webb is not able to have his bowels open after three days, and Margaret administers two glycerin suppositories which have effect with the minimum strain for Mr Webb.
Actual	Difficulty in re-establishing the pattern of micturition after the removal of the catheter on day 3 post-operatively.	Margaret explains to Mr Webb that his bladder muscle is like all muscle as it loses tone when not used. The presence of the catheter continuously draining urine has resulted in such loss of tone. This is quickly regained in the first day or two, but she tells him that he may only pass small amounts quite frequently until bladder tone returns. She explains the use of a Time and Amount chart to him on which he records the volume of urine passed at any one time, in order that his progress can be monitored. The internal sphincter in the bladder is damaged during prostatectomy, and patients therefore rely afterwards on external sphincter control, hence the reason for careful post-operative observation of the pattern of micturition.	Mr Webb is able to pass urine at lunchtime, although only 75 ml. He continues to pass volumes of not more than 170 ml approximately every two hours that day, and is up several times in the night. He is not concerned about his frequency, as Margaret had told him to expect this. By day 6 post-operatively he is passing 200–300 ml, every 3–4 hours, and is very pleased with the improvement the operation has made.

Bladder irrigation involves setting up a container of normal saline (0.9% sodium chloride) which runs from an infusion stand through tubing connected to the catheter. Via the catheter it runs into the bladder and out into the urine collection bag. Irrigation may be carried out continuously or intermittently. The decision about which is used depends upon the extent of surgery (and thus the degree of haemorrhage), and the surgeon's wishes. A two-way catheter will allow only for intermittent irrigation. A three-way catheter will allow for intermittent or continuous irrigation.

What should be done if the catheter appears blocked?
1 Ensure that the tubing is not kinked, and flow of irrigation impaired in any way.
2 Check the drainage tube into the collection bag for kinked tubing.
3 Milk the tubing, using catheter milkers.
4 Perform a bladder washout under strict aseptic conditions.

Irrigation that is well supervised should prevent catheter blockage!

Removal of catheters
Catheters should be removed preferably at the beginning of the day. This allows the patient a reasonable space of time in which to pass urine, so that, should re-catheterisation be required, it may be done in early evening to ensure that the patient is not uncomfortable all night. When removing catheters, the manufacturer's instructions should be followed. The water should be withdrawn from the balloon with a syringe, and then the catheter gently removed.

Post-operative haematuria is light, moderate or dark. Light haematuria is the colour of rosé wine. Moderate haematuria appears heavily blood-stained. Dark haematuria has the appearance of frank blood.

RETURNING HOME

Mr Webb has recovered well, and is eager to return to his wife, although she has been managing well in his absence. He leaves hospital for home after one week. Margaret ensures that he has medication for his chronic bronchitis. He does not need instructions regarding this, as he was taking the medication previously. He is advised to continue with a fluid intake of 1–2 litres per 24 hours, and eat a well-balanced diet to avoid constipation. He is told not to do any heavy work at home, or any lifting, until seen in the clinic in four weeks

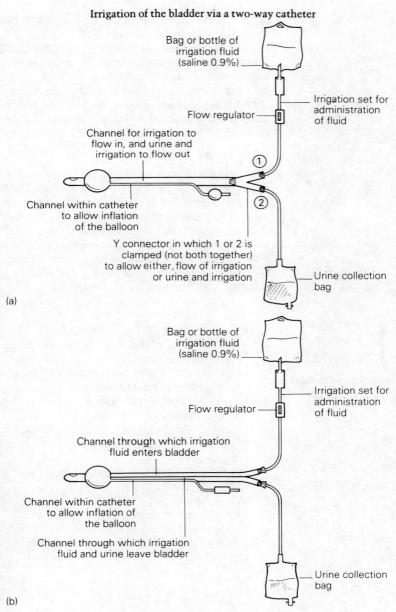

Irrigation of the bladder via a two-way catheter

Bag or bottle of irrigation fluid (saline 0.9%)

Irrigation set for administration of fluid

Flow regulator

Channel for irrigation to flow in, and urine and irrigation to flow out

①

②

Channel within catheter to allow inflation of the balloon

Y connector in which 1 or 2 is clamped (not both together) to allow either, flow of irrigation or urine and irrigation

Urine collection bag

(a)

Bag or bottle of irrigation fluid (saline 0.9%)

Irrigation set for administration of fluid

Flow regulator

Channel through which irrigation fluid enters bladder

Channel within catheter to allow inflation of the balloon

Channel through which irrigation fluid and urine leave bladder

Urine collection bag

(b)

Irrigation of the bladder via a three-way catheter

time, in order to avoid risk of haemorrhage until the tissues are well healed.

He has received a letter from his daughter in Australia inviting her mother and father again for a holiday, and saying that everything will be organised so that her mother can manage. As he feels so much better, he has decided that they should make the trip while they can, and is eager to get home to discuss it with his wife.

Note

The length of stay in hospital following this operation may be more or less than in Mr Webb's case, as it is variable in different hospitals. As many patients are elderly, however, it is important that their general state of health is considered, as well as the operation undergone. There are variations too in the person's ability to cope alone if home support is inadequate for the situation presented.

<table>
<tr><td>TEST YOURSELF</td><td>1</td><td>What were Mr Webb's symptoms?</td></tr>
<tr><td></td><td>2</td><td>Why did Mr Webb have a trans-urethral resection of prostate?</td></tr>
<tr><td></td><td>3</td><td>How did the nurse help Mr Webb to cope with epidural anaesthesia?</td></tr>
<tr><td></td><td>4</td><td>How did the nurse monitor Mr Webb's condition post-operatively?</td></tr>
<tr><td></td><td>5</td><td>Why did Mr Webb have bladder irrigation?</td></tr>
<tr><td></td><td>6</td><td>How did the nurses manage the bladder irrigation?</td></tr>
<tr><td></td><td>7</td><td>What nursing action was to be taken if the catheter ceased draining?</td></tr>
<tr><td></td><td>8</td><td>What were Mr Webb's feelings about nurses performing catheter hygiene?</td></tr>
<tr><td></td><td>9</td><td>What was important for the nurse to explain to Mr Webb when the catheter was removed?</td></tr>
</table>

FURTHER READING

Franklin, B. L. 1974. *Patient Anxiety on Admission to Hospital*. London: RCN.

Hayward, J. 1975. *Information: A Prescription Against Pain*. London: RCN.

Wright, L. 1974. *Bowel Function in Hospital Patients*. London: RCN.

8 Caring for a young patient who is undergoing testicular surgery

Errol James is a 14-year-old schoolboy who lives with his parents and two sisters. His mother is a nurse, and his father is a college lecturer. Errol has recently returned to school after spending the summer holiday with his grand-parents in the West Indies.

He is a very keen football player, and his ambition is to play professional football for a top club. He represents his school and his county in the under-15 team.

Whilst on the football field one afternoon practising with his team, he receives a severe kick to his scrotum whilst tackling for the ball. He is in severe pain following this incident, and is helped from the pitch. His injury is very painful, and his scrotum is becoming swollen. As a result of this, he is taken immediately to the Accident and Emergency department of the local hospital. On examination the doctor diagnoses torsion of the left testis. As this condition requires urgent surgical treatment, Errol's mother is contacted and arrives within half-an-hour to sign the consent form for his operation.

The doctor explains to Mrs James that it may be necessary to remove the testis if they find that lack of circulation has affected it too

Torsion of the testis

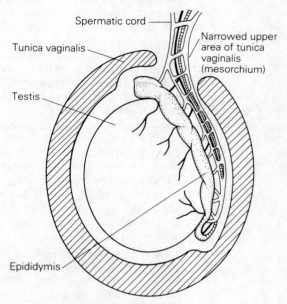

Spermatic cord

Narrowed upper
area of tunica
vaginalis
(mesorchium)

Tunica vaginalis

Testis

Epididymis

severely. Although the surgery is urgent, he is
admitted to the ward prior to surgery as there
is a short interval of time while essential
arrangements are made, and it is felt that Errol
may be less anxious than if he was sitting in
the Accident and Emergency department.

Torsion of the testis constitutes a surgical emergency.
The testis is suspended by mesentery (mesorchium), and
if this becomes twisted it interferes with the blood
supply. Uncorrected, gangrene may occur. This condition
is common around puberty, and can be caused by
congenital abnormality associated with undescended
testes, and also by trauma.

**INITIAL
NURSING
CARE**

Errol arrives on the ward accompanied by
his mother, and they are both welcomed by
Margaret, the ward nurse. Errol is helped into a
bed in a bay where there are several patients of
a similar age. Both Errol and his mother are
very anxious. He is obviously frightened about

the operation, and has been in considerable pain, although analgesia administered in the Accident and Emergency department has relieved this.

His mother is very anxious about the prospect of Errol having one testis removed. She is a midwife, and therefore understands the implications of this operation and its possible effects on his future fertility.

Margaret reassures Errol that the operation will be over very quickly, and that he will soon be able to play sport again. She explains that, after the operation, he will have to rest in bed for a day, and will probably feel very sore. She assures him that analgesia will be given for his pain. (Such information improves post-operative pain; Hayward 1975). Margaret offers Mrs James a cup of tea, and while she is drinking this, Margaret carries out a series of baseline observations of TPR and BP and urinalysis, all of which are within normal limits. She explains to Errol that he will require a pubic shave, but in view of the urgency this will be carried out in theatre. He is very relieved at this, as he would find it very embarrassing.

He has just passed urine, and is therefore helped into an operation gown by his mother and settled in the bed. After placing an identiband on his wrist and ensuring that he is not wearing any jewellery, he is given premedication which he is told will make him drowsy and make his mouth feel dry. He has not eaten for four hours, and it will therefore be safe for him to have an anaesthetic.

Margaret escorts Errol to theatre, and, on her return, his father has arrived. She is able to refer both parents to the ward sister who spends further time discussing the situation, which eases some of their anxiety, particularly with regard to Errol's future fertility. A left orchidectomy is indicated. (Now refer to the Nursing Care Plan for Errol.)

Orchidectomy is the surgical removal of the testis.

Post-operative Nursing Care Plan for Errol

PROBLEM	NATURE	NURSING CARE AND RATIONALE	EVALUATION
Actual	Pain and discomfort due to a surgical incision and a swollen scrotum.	Analgesia is given as prescribed, and is given regularly to ensure Errol's pain is kept under control. He is not wearing a wound dressing, as the wound has been sprayed with 'plastic skin' (e.g. Nobecutane), but is wearing a scrotal support which helps to relieve the discomfort of a swollen scrotum. Margaret ensures that he remains on bed rest for the first day to minimise swelling and consequent damage to the other testis. She places a bed cradle in the bed to keep the weight of the bedclothes from Errol's pelvis.	Errol is happy to stay in bed that first day, listening to the radio and looking at magazines. As his pain is well relieved, however, he is pleased to be allowed up the following day.
Actual	Embarrassment at having to use a urinal in the initial post-operative period, and at having his wound site observed by the nursing staff.	Margaret tries to do as much as possible for Errol, as she has already established a rapport with him, having admitted him. He is particularly vulnerable to this form of embarrassment at the age of 14 years, and all the nurses try to give him as much privacy as possible and preserve his dignity. His mother helps him a good deal with personal hygiene, and this minimises his embarrassment.	By showing empathy for his feelings, Margaret and her colleagues are able to help Errol to feel less embarrassed.

Post-operative Nursing Care Plan for Errol

PROBLEM	NATURE	NURSING CARE AND RATIONALE	EVALUATION
Potential	Infection of the wound due to its position on the scrotum.	The wound site is protected by 'plastic skin' which prevents contamination with micro-organisms and from splashes of urine. Margaret and Errol's mother observe the site for signs of inflammation, increased swelling, or discharge. Errol is encouraged to be particularly careful about personal hygiene around the penis and scrotum, to prevent contamination of the area with micro-organisms.	Errol is reluctant to wash too vigorously around the area, as he is frightened of any discomfort it may cause, but with adequate analgesia and explanation he manages well. The sutures are of an absorbable variety, and so Errol is spared the discomfort and embarrassment of them having to be removed.
Actual	Restricted mobility due to scrotal swelling.	Errol is encouraged to mobilise gently, once the first day of bed rest is over. He is keen to watch TV, and this is an incentive to walk to the dayroom. Margaret suggests short frequent walks, and his parents help and encourage him.	Errol gradually increases his degree of mobility, and as he finds the scrotal support uncomfortable, a snug-fitting pair of underpants are used instead. These make him more comfortable and he increases his level of activity.

Errol is discharged four days after his operation. He is reassured that, cosmetically, it is not obvious that he now has only one testis. He and his parents are told that his other testis is quite normal.

The parents and Errol are all concerned about his future sporting activities and his dream of becoming a professional footballer, but he is told that this should not make any difference to his lifestyle, only that he should wear appropriate scrotal protection for sport in future.

Errol is also advised to wear swimming trunks under his clothes for several weeks, as these would provide him with added scrotal support. He is given an outpatient appointment for four weeks, and advised not to play football or other sport until then to allow complete healing of the wound.

**TEST
YOURSELF**

1 Why did Errol develop torsion of the testis?
2 What was the nurse's role in explaining his operation to him?
3 What care and support did the nurse give to Errol's parents?
4 Why did Errol have an orchidectomy?
5 How did the nurse minimise Errol's embarrassment when delivering care?
6 What important advice did Errol receive on returning home?

**FURTHER
READING**

Hayward, J. 1975. *Information: A Prescription Against Pain*. London: RCN.

9

Caring for a patient who is undergoing urinary diversion

HISTORY

Mrs Evelyn Simpson is a 55-year-old lady who helps her husband to run his butcher's shop. She has always been an active lady, having had three children and always helped in her husband's business. She also has a hobby of flower-arranging, and enters many competitions. She is an active gardener, providing the raw materials for her hobby. Mrs Simpson's other favourite pastime is swimming, and she helps a group of disabled people every week when they have swimming sessions at the local baths.

Ten years ago, Mrs Simpson was diagnosed as having carcinoma of the bladder, for which she has had regular check cystoscopies and treatment of any recurrence. Unfortunately, in the past three years the disease has progressed and resulted in discomfort and unpleasant symptoms of haematuria, infections, dysuria and frequency. In spite of radiotherapy treatment, the disease is now extensive, and Mrs Simpson is very distressed at its effect on her life, and she does not wish to continue with such a miserable lifestyle. After discussions in the Outpatient Department, Mrs Simpson is admitted with a view to having a urinary diversion performed.

Urinary diversion involves diverting the urine away from the bladder. It may be performed not only for bladder tumours, but also for chronic incontinence involving totally inadequate bladder control, and, in children, for congenital abnormalities of the urinary system. Urinary diversion takes two forms:

1 Ureterosigmoidostomy
This is often referred to as 'rectal bladder', in which the ureters are diverted to drain into the sigmoid colon, rather than the bladder. This results in the patient passing urine and faeces per rectum. Its disadvantages are that, as the main function of the colon is water absorption, electrolyte imbalance may result from reabsorption of urine. Kidney infection and subsequent septicaemia are a problem because *Escherichia coli* is normal flora to the large intestine, and the most common infective organism of the urinary tract. The patient is also always passing what appears to be 'diarrhoea' – urine and faeces mixed. The major advantage is that the patient's external appearance is, in principle, unchanged.

2 Ileal conduit
This is more commonly performed, and involves diversion of the ureters from the bladder to a piece of ileum – separated from the small bowel but still attached to its mesentery – which forms a stoma brought out on to the skin surface, and allowing urine to drain into an appliance or 'bag' on the surface of the abdomen (see p. 78).

The formation of an ileal conduit

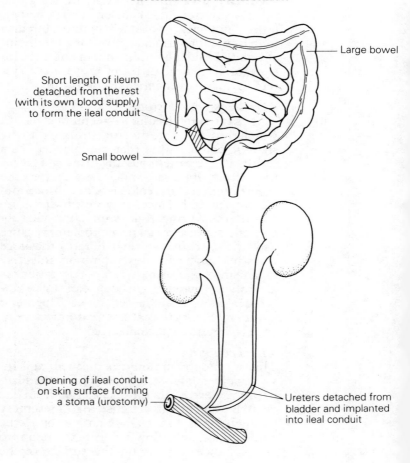

Short length of ileum detached from the rest (with its own blood supply) to form the ileal conduit

Small bowel

Large bowel

Opening of ileal conduit on skin surface forming a stoma (urostomy)

Ureters detached from bladder and implanted into ileal conduit

After further discussion with the surgeons it is agreed with Mrs Simpson that she will have an ileal conduit formed. (Refer now to the Nursing Care Plans for Mrs Simpson.)

Pre-operative Nursing Care Plan for Mrs Simpson

ACTUAL PROBLEM	NURSING CARE AND RATIONALE	EVALUATION
Concern, anxiety and embarrassment about the prospect of wearing 'a bag' to collect urine, although she is desperate for relief of her symptoms.	Mrs Simpson is allowed every opportunity to discuss her concerns and, where necessary, Margaret arranges further discussions with the doctor for her. She and her husband are introduced to the stoma care specialist nurse, who is able to discuss their concerns and provide answers to many questions. Wherever possible, Margaret joins in to enable her to provide ongoing support for her patient. Mrs Simpson is introduced to another patient who had this operation several years previously and is fit and well.	Many of Mrs Simpson's questions are answered by the stoma nurse, medical staff and the other patient. Although she is understandably anxious, she is much more at ease.
Mrs Simpson is concerned about what she considers to be a loss of femininity or altered body image, as she feels this will affect her husband's attitude towards her.	Mrs Simpson needs time to come to terms with the proposed alteration in her body image. She is offered every opportunity for discussion, and the stoma care nurse is particularly well qualified to counsel her. She is assured that sexual relations with her husband need not be affected by this surgery. Margaret encourages Mrs Simpson to ask questions, and arranges for her to see other staff as necessary. She also encourages her to include Mr Simpson in as much discussion as possible.	This problem cannot be resolved overnight, and Mr and Mrs Simpson will work through their difficulties together. They are a close couple, and, with the counselling support, will jointly plan to help Mrs Simpson come to terms with the change.

Pre-operative Nursing Care Plan for Mrs Simpson

ACTUAL PROBLEM	NURSING CARE AND RATIONALE	EVALUATION
The position of the stoma is a concern to Mrs Simpson, as she feels the bag may prevent her from continuing her active lifestyle, and thus cause her embarrassment.	Prior to operation, the stoma care nurse marks the site for the stoma on Mrs Simpson's abdomen. This ensures that the stoma will not be situated in skin folds where a bag cannot be easily fixed; Mrs Simpson's usual clothing, activities and hobbies are all discussed before the site is chosen.	Mrs Simpson is heartened by the fact that she can still wear her swimsuit, and by the advice and information about various items of clothing now manufactured which will disguise her appliance.
Mrs Simpson's bowel is loaded with faeces and needs to be empty prior to surgery.	Margaret explains carefully to Mrs Simpson that, as the operation involves both the gastro-intestinal and urinary systems, it is essential for the bowel to be as empty as possible to facilitate the operation, and reduce possible contamination of the operation site. Mrs Simpson therefore takes strong oral aperients and is allowed fluids only for 24 hours prior to the operation. She is then not allowed anything by mouth four hours before her operation (Hamilton-Smith 1972) to avoid the possibility of regurgitation or inhalation of vomit.	Mrs Simpson's aperients have an excellent result, although it involves several trips to the toilet for her. She manages to tolerate fluids only, although finds it difficult when other patients are eating, and goes to sit in the dayroom at mealtimes.

Mrs Simpson is concerned about the post-operative period, and how soon she will be up and about.

Margaret explains that, as both the gastro-intestinal and urinary systems will be operated upon, they will both require care after the operation. She explains that Mrs Simpson will return to the ward with a naso-gastric tube *in situ*. Peristalsis of the gastro-intestinal tract ceases when it is handled at operation, and sometimes takes several days to return, hence the need to aspirate gastric juices in the interim. Nothing is given orally at this time. Mrs Simpson is also informed by Margaret that she will have an IVI to hydrate her in the absence of an oral fluid intake. She will have an abdominal wound and drain, as well as her stoma. Margaret is able to reassure her that she will be out of bed, even if only for short periods, within the first two days.

Mrs Simpson feels well prepared for her operation, having some idea of what to expect afterwards.

Post-operative Nursing Care Plan for Mrs Simpson

PROBLEM	NATURE	NURSING CARE AND RATIONALE	EVALUATION
Actual	Pain and discomfort due to an abdominal incision.	Margaret ensures that analgesia is given as prescribed, and a comfortable position obtained by positioning pillows to give Mrs Simpson adequate support both when sitting up and lying down.	Pain is minimised by the regular analgesia and a comfortable position.
Actual	Mrs Simpson finds the naso-gastric tube rather uncomfortable.	The tube is positioned so as not to cause undue pressure on the nostrils, and not to obstruct the field of vision when fixed to the forehead. Margaret ensures that Mrs Simpson's nostrils are kept clean, and that tape used to secure the tube is used sparingly and kept clear of surrounding hair. The tube is aspirated gently according to the volumes of aspirate obtained, but, initially, every half-hour. Margaret leaves the tube on free drainage in the interim, to ensure no build-up of fluid which might make Mrs Simpson feel nauseous. She ensures that all aspirate is measured and recorded on the fluid-balance chart.	Although the tube is not pleasant, careful management enables Mrs Simpson to tolerate it for the required 2–3 days.

Actual	Mrs Simpson has a dry mouth, due to restriction of oral fluids.	Margaret offers her frequent mouthwashes, and she is allowed 30 ml of water orally each hour (or ice to suck) to moisten the oral mucosa. This is given after aspiration, to avoid it being aspirated back immediately. All oral fluid is recorded on the fluid-balance chart.	Mrs Simpson's oral mucosa is kept moist, and she feels quite comfortable.
Potential	Mrs Simpson may become dehydrated without oral fluids.	Margaret monitors the IVI which is *in situ*, ensuring that it runs at the correct rate, so that Mrs Simpson receives the correct amount of fluids to avoid dehydration. All IV fluids are recorded on the fluid-balance chart.	Mrs Simpson remains well-hydrated and comfortable while oral fluid is restricted, and she commences an increased fluid intake, progressing to free fluids after three days. Her IVI is then discontinued.
Actual	Mrs Simpson now has a urinary stoma for drainage of urine.	Margaret observes the stoma whenever she carries out other observations. This is to ensure that the stoma is healthy, indicated by pink mucosa, and that the position of the stoma is correct. This would not be the case if the stoma were dusky in colour (indicating poor blood supply) or bright red (indicating inflammation). If the stoma were barely visible, or appeared to have prolapsed, this should be reported to the nurse in charge immediately, so that it can be sutured in position again. The stoma nurse is supportive of Margaret and the other nurses in caring for the stoma.	Mrs Simpson's stoma is pink and healthy, and drains good volumes of urine which Margaret records on the fluid balance chart.

Post-operative Nursing Care Plan for Mrs Simpson

PROBLEM	NATURE	NURSING CARE AND RATIONALE	EVALUATION
Actual	Mrs Simpson's mobility is impaired, due to her recent major abdominal operation.	Mrs Simpson is encouraged by Margaret to avoid possible problems arising from the impaired mobility. She is encouraged to perform leg exercises, and sits out of bed for increasing periods from the first post-operative day to minimise the risk of deep vein thrombosis formation. Margaret assists her with deep breathing exercises, giving her advice about how to support her abdomen when doing these. The physiotherapist also encourages Mrs Simpson with her deep breathing exercises. Margaret also assists Mrs Simpson with personal hygiene.	With adequate analgesia prior to washing and mobilising, Mrs Simpson is able to avoid any complications of impaired mobility.

Actual	Mrs Simpson has to learn how to manage her new stoma.	In the initial post-operative period, Margaret and the other nurses, together with the stoma care nurse, empty and change the urinary appliance as necessary, ensuring that the skin is well protected so as to prevent contact with urine and subsequent excoriation. Under the supervision of the nurses, Mrs Simpson is encouraged in subsequent days to accept her stoma by beginning to care for it. Where possible, her husband is encouraged to be present in order that his support and acceptance can give encouragement to her. Initially, Mrs Simpson is shown how to empty the bag, and, having become proficient at this, is taught how to change appliances.	Mrs Simpson learns very quickly, in spite of feeling initial anxiety. She is greatly helped by her husband's support. By day 6 post-operatively she is able to empty the bag herself, and by day 9, change it completely.
Potential	Infection of the wound, and urinary infection.	Margaret observes the wound for signs of redness, swelling or discharge, which could indicate infection. She also observes drainage from the wound drain for signs of purulence, and records the volume of output on the fluid-balance chart. Margaret maintains observations of temperature and pulse every four hours, as, if these are raised, it could indicate infection. Stoma care is carried out carefully to minimise infection (although this is a clean, not aseptic procedure). Mrs Simpson is encouraged to have an oral intake of 2–3 litres per day to ensure good renal filtration and urine output.	The wound heals well, the drain being removed after three days, and the sutures after 10 days. Mrs Simpson's urine remains free of infection.

RETURNING HOME

Mrs Simpson makes an uneventful recovery, and is managing her stoma well. She is discharged on day 12 post-operatively. The stoma care nurse assures her that she will keep in touch, and gives her a telephone number where she can be contacted if any difficulties arise. She ensures that Mrs Simpson knows how to obtain new supplies of appliances which are available on prescription.

Mrs Simpson is given the address of the Urinary Conduit Association of which she can become a member if she wishes. It could provide a contact for her with other people having urinary stomas.

She is advised not to return to working in the butcher's shop for a month, until seen again at the Outpatient Clinic. This time will enable her abdominal tissues to heal fully. She is reassured, however, that, after attending the clinic, she can gradually return to her work and to her hobbies of flower-arranging and swimming. She is looking forward to an improved quality of life with her husband and family now that she has the ileal conduit.

If she becomes concerned about further complications in the future, and her overall prognosis, a session with the surgeon could be arranged.

TEST YOURSELF

1 Why did Mrs Simpson require an ileal conduit?
2 What were Mrs Simpson's feelings about the operation?
3 How did the team explain the surgery and its consequences to Mrs Simpson?
4 Why was it important to restrict gastrointestinal activity for this surgery?
5 How was Mrs Simpson helped to overcome her embarrassment and fears about her new body image?

6 Why was skin care and observation of the stoma an important aspect of post-operative nursing care?

7 How was Mrs Simpson helped to learn to care for her stoma, by both the stoma care nurse and the ward nurse?

8 Prior to Mrs Simpson's return home, what help and information can the nursing team provide to ensure that she is successful in returning to a full life?

FURTHER READING

Hamilton-Smith, S. 1972. *Nil by Mouth? A Descriptive Study of Nursing Care in Relation to Pre-operative Fasting*. London: RCN.

Edwards, S. 1984. The fashioning of an ileal conduit. *Nursing Mirror* (16 May 1984), **158**(20), 35–37.

Lawson, A. 1979. Ileal conduit. *Nursing Times*, supplement on Community Outlook, 8th March 1979.

Lawson, A. 1980. *Understanding Urostomy*. Squibb Surgicare Ltd.

10 Conclusion

This short text has not been able to provide you with care studies of patients with every type of urinary problem or disease that you may meet on the genito-urinary ward.

You will encounter patients with malignant disease who, while requiring surgery and the kind of care outlined in the preceding chapters, will also require other nursing skills. They may have to undergo radiotherapy or chemotherapy, and need much psychological as well as specific physical care.

As you are new to the specialty, you can seek support and guidance from senior members of staff to help you care for these patients.

In this ward you will also meet patients undergoing various types of reconstructive surgery, and, again, senior nurses will guide you and share their knowledge and expertise with you when caring for such patients.

In summary, the care studies in this book should provide you with sound guidelines in order that you can provide a high standard of care for patients with genito-urinary problems.

It is important to remember that many patients endure urinary problems in the community (e.g. cystitis and incontinence). You may not see these patients in the ward at all, or only when their conditions become complicated or more serious. You may, of course, see them when you visit in the community, and some of the information thus gained may prove of use to you.

In the genito-urinary ward there are many

changes and advances relating to nursing care, for example, the innovations in equipment and appliances for incontinent patients. It is important to update your knowledge in order that you are better able to advise patients, and thus improve their quality of life.

New technology is having far-reaching effects on genito-urinary medicine and surgery, and this, in turn, may affect the type of nursing care required by your patients (e.g. lithotripsy).

In conclusion, it is hoped that you, as the reader and carer, will have developed an increased awareness of the anxiety and embarrassment endured, often unnecessarily, by many patients.

People are entitled to the highest level of care that we can provide. People with genito-urinary problems have special problems, perhaps many months of discomfort, pain and embarrassment. This can have great effect on a person's life quality. We as nurses have a responsibility to maintain and enhance our skills and knowledge in relation to all aspects of a person's care.